"You don't get MS until you GET MS"
- Anonymous

"I just might have a problem
That you'll understand
We all need somebody to lean on"
- Lean on Me Lyrics by Bill Withers

"To be beautiful means to be yourself. You don't
need to be accepted by others. You need to accept
yourself.'
- Thich Nhat Hạnh

"In three words, I can completely describe to you
what I've learned about life – It goes on."
- Robert Frost

It's Not as Bad as it Sounds

Cover Illustration: "Flirtation"
 (by Yvonne Decelis)

I am NOT a Doctor or a Physician. I am a patient
and everything written here is written from my
own experience(s). If you are in need of medical
assistance please contact a health
care professional.

Email: YDCBook@yahoo.com
Facebook: https://www.facebook.com/ydcbook

v.9   8-Mar-14
v.10 11-Nov-14

TABLE OF CONTENTS

It's Not as Bad as it Sounds

Thrill Ride (*by Yvonne Decelis*)

It's a slow rollercoaster
Every day
I feel my brain peel away
Now...
Layer by layer
Piece by piece
It's much smaller
Now...
Then it was
Fifteen years ago
Everything is
A little harder to do
Now...
Then it was
Ten years ago
Five years ago
Yesterday
This morning
Now...

Yvonne Decelis

Acknowledgements

I have many people to thank so I am going to start this off by apologizing in advance if your name is not listed here and it should be. My short-term memory is HORRIBLE. If you are not on here and you should be, please let me know and I will be sure to mention you in my next book or any new editions that may come from this one.

I want to start this off by thanking the two most important (in my opinion) people in my life: my husband and my mother. The two of you have kept me strong through all of the storm clouds I have been through. Your love and understanding has meant the world to me and I honestly do not know how I would have survived without you in my life. I also want to thank a very good friend and neighbor, Alicia Dasilva. Alicia, you gave me friendship, love, guidance and encouragement (and a VERY cool nickname – possibly the coolest nickname anyone has ever given me, "V") at a time when I needed it very badly. I thank you very much for everything and for being there!

I also need to mention a good friend, a former classmate and a fellow writer from the University of Massachusetts (UMass), James (who I know as Jimmy) Murphy. Jimmy – you really are just like a brother to me and I love you like family. When I found out I was going to be in a class with a Vietnam era Veteran I was honored. I have been fascinated with Vietnam ever since reading some of the books by Timothy Obrien (the first one I read being The Things They Carried). Thank you so much for being there for me Jimmy, and thank you for all of your encouragement!

I have to thank ALL of the teachers I had while I was at Umass Boston's College of Public and Community Service. In particular, I want to thank Nina Silverstein, Raul Ybarra, Andrew Leong, Michael Stone, Ann Withorn, Fadia Harik and Luis Aponte-Parés. I have always loved writing, but you all helped me to develop extra confidence in myself (in my capabilities as a writer, a public speaker, a citizen and a scholar). Many of the students who I attended CPCS with also helped my self-confidence (dramatically). In the interest of time, suffice it to say that I do not know that I could have done this without all of you.

I also want to thank my Neurologist at Brigham and Women's' Hospital, Dr. Maria Houtchens. Dr. Houtchens, you have been the best Neurologist I have had so far (throughout this bumpy ride). You are down to earth and you do not "speak down" to me. I could also tell that you were completely sincere when you told me how proud you were of how I was doing in school. That sincerity meant and continues to mean a lot to me. You are a wonderful doctor and a great person and I consider you to be a friend, something I cannot say for many other doctors that I have had in the past.

I am also going to use this section to make a mention of Stan Swartz, a very good friend of mine who has an online support group called Stan's Angels (http://www.stansangels.com/). I elaborate more about Stan in the section about "Thing's I'm Grateful for". Suffice it to say (for now) that I owe a lot of thanks to Stan and to the many Angels who have signed up for his support group (quite a few of these people are very close friends and some are like family). The people who are members of this support group are people who have MS (and/or people who know them).

Reading stories from "like-minded" individuals who know what I go through on a day-to-day basis along with forming these friendships has really helped inspire me to do this book. Thank you so much to every single one of you!

Last but definitely not least, I need to bring up the gratitude I have for people no longer on "this mortal coil" that I feel I, at the very least, owe a mention to. My stepfather, Martin Blatz (he was a true inspiration to me. He was brilliant and a man of grace and style); my grandmother Sylvia (I thank her for being all that she was and for reuniting me with my father. I miss my stepfather and grandmother so much. I don't think you can ever truly "get over" losing a loved one. The pain just ebbs away – eventually but not completely); my grandfather and great Aunt; and two very good friends of mine who died LONG before their time, Elizabeth Hardenbergh and Emanuel Pimentel (I can not put into words how much I miss you both. Your deaths were complete shocks to me and I will never forget you).

Introduction

My "journey" with Multiple Sclerosis (MS) and Fibromyalgia (Fibro) is about going through the diagnosis process and living with both "invisible illnesses". I am writing this to help others avoid and/or expect the pitfalls that I have stumbled across. I am also hopeful that this will help people find ways to help themselves. Last but not least, I want to make sure others who have a desire to learn what makes us "tick" will come away from this having learned things that will help them and us, the patients.

By the way – I often refer to us (people in the disabled community) as patients throughout this book. Please know I am not doing this to define us. Just because we have these invisible conditions many assume that it is OK to think of us as patients and nothing more. I am here to state that we are MUCH more than that.

Who is this book for? I have been asked who I see as my "target" audience for this book. As with life, there is no easy answer to that question. I am primarily writing this for people afflicted with Multiple Sclerosis, Fibromyalgia, or any other illness that makes this book relatable to them.

It's Not as Bad as it Sounds

However, I am also writing this book for people who know others with these conditions, for people in the medical industry, and/or for anyone who just want to know more. No matter who you are, if you are reading this then chances are good that this is for you.

I will be thanking you quite a bit throughout this book but to start things off right I want to thank you for taking the time and having an interest in reading this to begin with. Knowledge is power and one problem many of us often come across is an almost willful ignorance about the things we have to face and go through every day. In getting this book you have taken a very important first step and for that you deserve a lot of gratitude. I thank you again; this really means more to me than I can express.

If you are a patient the first thing I want to say is that I am very sorry for what you are going through. NOBODY deserves to suffer and it breaks my heart every time I hear of a new diagnosis being given out. I am sorry for what you are going through and I want you to know you are not alone. I truly hope you can come away from reading this with an at least slightly more positive/hopeful outlook about whatever you are going through.

It's Not as Bad as it Sounds

There are some basic logistics that I would like to add before we get started: Most of the names I use in this book have been changed. If you see yourself in any of the more negative things I write about please do not assume I mean you, even if we know each other, even if you are absolutely certain I mean you. I only use real names for people I have had positive experiences with and, even then, some names may be changed to protect peoples' privacy.

In addition, if you read this from start-to-finish you are going to see a lot of repeated sentences and/or themes (for example, I am NOT a medical Professional). This (redundancy) is not because I am looking down on you or because I need "filler material" or anything like that. Part of it is because these chapters were written at different times over the past couple of years. Another reason is because I want each section to stand on its own as much as possible. The last reason for some of the repetition is likely to be my own faulty short-term memory.

My MS (and Fibro) "Journey"

I was diagnosed with Relapsing Remitting Multiple Sclerosis (MS) in December of 1994. While I thought this news was devastating, I was relieved to find out things weren't much worse. In February of 1993, I went to the Hospital for what I thought was an odd bout of conjunctivitis (AKA pink eye). I realized how wrong I was when the doctor looked at me and then went to get five or six of his "colleagues".

They all looked at me and spoke as if I was not there (in third person). My symptoms were that, whenever I looked at something diagonally, my vision would double and get blurry. I also found out my pupils were two different sizes from hearing the doctors discuss me. I felt like a lab rat. They may have well referred to me as an "it" – that is exactly how they made me feel.

Eventually, I was informed (in a very "matter-of-fact" tone) that I might have a brain tumor and that there were no magnetic resonance imaging (MRI) machines available. I had to go in the following day. To "ease the news" for me I was told that I had classic stroke symptoms and that I was fortunate they were not testing me for one. He said those tests were more intrusive and/or harmful than anything I would need to endure. Despite the assurances that I was very fortunate that these dangerous exams were not going to be performed on me, I was very shaken up by what I considered to be a bombshell that had just been dropped on me.

The ride home on the subway from this appointment was awful; it was impossible for me not to cry in public over what I had just found out. A man to my left asked if I needed help and I shook my head no. He then loudly said to the girl with him "oh sure, nothing's wrong. She's sitting there crying but oh no, nothing's wrong with her!'" At the following stop, I jumped out to get into another trolley car but on the way past I got close to him and said, "I got on the train at a hospital stop. Put two and two together you idiot!"

My first MRI was a horrifying experience for me. I was asked if I was claustrophobic (to which I answered, "no.") For anyone who has ever had an MRI (in a body-length MRI tube) this may not sound too unfamiliar to relate to. I remember thinking later that asking if someone is claustrophobic is not a good enough way to find out how they will do in an MRI tube. However, I suppose asking someone if they could handle spending an hour in a tube with a cage around their head might scare them off worse. However, I had never had an MRI before and therefore had no idea what I was about to go through.

About halfway through the MRI I had a panic/anxiety attack and had to be sedated. I remember not being able to move my arms and thinking about my grandmother's entombment (and thinking the opening to the tube was going to be closed off). Unlike most MRI machines I have been in recently, this first one was in a "full body" tube. It was a horrible introduction to the experience.

I do not want to make MRIs sound worse than they are. I have come a long way from that first MRI experience. I fall asleep during the scans now. During my first scan, I wound up having to come out for a bit from the extremely closed-in sensation (in addition to the unbelievably loud sounds the machine made. In a lot of places they may not warn you about that. It is incredibly loud because the sound is right by your head, which intensifies the volume level).

The results came in about 3 days after I had the scan. I was told I might have Multiple Sclerosis (MS) or Lupus but the doctors were really not certain. I was told it could be nothing but not to discount the possibility that something was wrong. Despite this I managed to put the entire ordeal almost completely out of my mind for about a year following.

Now I am going to fast forward a bit in the interest of not wanting to make your eyes bleed. I appreciate you taking the time to read this so I will refrain from babbling as much as I can. In an effort to be succinct, I will be skipping many details but I will fill them in as I am able.

In December of 1994, I had a new problem that I could not figure out how to explain to the Doctor who I went to see (I have since realized that my MS "attacks" are often very difficult to put into words). I knew it was a visual problem. Things looked blurry and if I turned to look sideways everything doubled and tripled up. Thankfully, at this point in my life I had health insurance so I was able to see a Primary Care Physician (PCP). I was then sent to see an eye doctor who conducted an exam called a visual field test on me. After the exam, he told me I needed to have an MRI.

This news did not make me very happy. It brought the incidents from the following year back to my memory. Thankfully, the second MRI I had was nowhere near as bad as the first one. In two days, I got the results while I was sitting at my desk at work. It was extremely difficult being told I probably had Multiple Sclerosis (once again) over the phone.

It was also a very frightening thing to find out it was very likely that I had MS. I knew absolutely nothing about Multiple Sclerosis when I first found out I had it. I thought it meant that any morning I could wake up unable to move. My biggest fear was the idea of waking up with no feelings from the neck down. The first Neurologist I had did absolutely nothing to assuage my fear. Now before you read this, please bear in mind that this Neurologist did not know what he was talking about (with regards to Multiple Sclerosis). I cannot bear the idea of another newly diagnosed patient reading this blatant misinformation and becoming frightened by it.

This Neurologist told me about a patient he had who came to him saying that her left arm and leg were tingling. He then told me that she quickly lost all feeling in one side of her body. I had no idea that this Doctor was using a very bad example since MS was something I still knew very little about. My mother was at this appointment with me, and this doctor managed to terrify both of us with his thoughtless comparison.

It's Not as Bad as it Sounds

Thankfully I was able to find a new Neurologist who specialized in working with MS patients and he was able to completely calm both my mother and me down. Unfortunately, for the first few years after my diagnosis I had a few exacerbations (aka MS Attacks or flares) at a rate of approximately one per year. The first two were bouts of Optic Neuritis; the first one being the strange eye trouble I had before being diagnosed. The second was a small blind spot in the same exact location for both eyes. I then had an attack that affected my mobility.

The last (and worst) MS attack I had was when I lost all feeling in my left arm. Being left-handed, this caused a lot of trouble for me. Even though I have had almost full recovery from the MS Attacks there were residual side effects from all of them (such as, but not limited to, balance trouble, vision issues, numbness and tingling, etc.) I cannot write more than a sentence without it hurting a great deal and my handwriting and signature both have changed quite a bit. Typing hurts after a while but thankfully I am able to do a bit of that. It really stinks not being able to write and I hope I can continue to type for as long as possible.

This last attack was in 1998. In 1999 I learned about Montel Williams being diagnosed with MS and I started to follow his progress. I am really glad

It's Not as Bad as it Sounds

I did as it helped me help myself. When I read about his athleticism, which I could see for myself when seeing him on TV, I decided I was going to do whatever it took to fight the "MonSter" (as many of us "MSers" refer to it online).

As much as I hate having this condition it was truly a "wake-up call" for me. Thanks to me deciding to become athletic I eventually quit smoking (over nine years ago as of now) and developed an almost religious workout regimen. As far as the exercise goes I am in slightly better shape now than I was when I was in my teens.

Please keep in mind that at this point in my life I am certain I was born with Multiple Sclerosis since I have always had a lot of health problems that only MS would explain. For example, my mother informed me that I have had a tremor ever since I was an infant. I remember finding a baby book she had about me and I was astounded at how often I was ill. It really seemed like I was in the hospital about 75% of the time. I also remember thinking I was amazed that my constant health problems did not give her a nervous breakdown.

Once again, I plan to skip some sections of my life so I can bring you to the point where I found out I also had Fibromyalgia. Multiple Sclerosis can cause very painful symptoms like spasticity pain. There is another problem called an "MS Hug" which, in my opinion, should have a different name. "Hug" makes it sound almost pleasant and nothing could be further from the truth. It feels like a corset is getting very tight (understatement) around the torso or, as another MS patient once said, it feels like the torso is being held and crushed by a gigantic gorilla. It is not unheard of for a patient experiencing a "hug" to think they are having a heart attack. It makes it hard to breath and can sometimes cause discomfort on one side of the body.

I didn't start experiencing the MS pains until after my attack in 1998. Unfortunately once they began

Yvonne Decelis

the pain troubles just kept getting worse. After being laid off from a job I had for almost twelve years the pain became unbearable. The reason for this was likely to be stress, but it also had to do with my workout schedule being "interrupted" for a brief period. A few years after I was let go, my stepfather passed away. When this happened my mother and I became much closer and I found out she might have Fibromyalgia. I had heard about Fibromyalgia but didn't know much about it. I certainly hadn't considered the possibility that I might have it as well. However, since I knew people who had Fibromyalgia and who had relatives with MS, I thought I should look into finding out if I had it too.

It's Not as Bad as it Sounds

In order to get my first diagnosis for Fibromyalgia (and after some extensive research on the subject), I went to a Rheumatologist. In my opinion, the first doctor I went to see was not the best I have ever been to. He didn't really take anything I had to say very seriously and he mocked me for a few things I had on my pill list. When he saw that I was taking Glucosamine he said "and what is this for? To benefit the manufacturer?" I kept my mouth shut but was pretty insulted by this (I was very tempted to ask him which pharmaceutical company was "padding his pockets" to make him ask such a thing but I did not).

He then suggested I take sleeping pills. I told him I could not understand why he thought I needed them. I explained that one of the worst day-to-day problems I had was never feeling awake and he said he felt I was not getting "restorative" sleep hence the sleeping pill suggestion, which I ignored. Let me correct that and state that I did once try a sedative before going to sleep - a very small dose of one and not even the full pill. As I feared, it completely knocked me out and I felt tired and much more fatigued than usual the following day so I never took one again. He also never really answered my question as to whether or not I had Fibro (actually his exact answer was "yeah, probably" accompanied by a shrug) but I later discovered that he put into my medical record that I had "mild Fibromyalgia" which turned out to be incorrect. I recently took a "trigger point" test and was told my Fibro was severe. He did not tell me this but thankfully my Neurologist did. Considering the way the former Rheumatologist treated me, the idea of him not diagnosing me properly did not surprise me.

Thankfully one of my MS friends told me about something called Low Dose Naltrexone (LDN) but I was never able to get a clear handle on what this drug was or what it would be good for. After I found out about the Fibromyalgia I decided to ask my Neurologist about it since I was having so much pain trouble that I was on a running dose of acetaminophen and oxycodone, something I was very unhappy about having to rely on.

Ironically enough, my mother had met another woman with Fibromyalgia who told her all about LDN. With the help of another MS friend, I learned how to obtain and use LDN. My Neurologist was unable to give me a script for LDN because the Hospital network that she was in did not consider it to be "real medicine".

I am still relatively new to the world of Fibromyalgia even though I think I may have had it for at least ten years. I had symptoms that Fibro would explain long before I was diagnosed with it. If you want to learn more about it, I recommend the following web page by the National Institute of Arthritis and Musculoskeletal and Skin Diseases (NIAMS) called Questions and Answers About Fibromyalgia at:

http://tinyurl.com/nwz9f6t

In my opinion, this web page is a very good source for anyone who wants to know more about this condition.

One final note about Fibromyalgia. Since I have had several people tell me that Fibro is a "BS condition" I wanted to provide this information I found on WebMD: ""Fibromyalgia may be related to a global dysfunction of cerebral pain-processing," study author Eric Guedj, MD, of Centre Hospitalo-Universitaire de la Timone, in Marseille, France, says in a news release. "This study demonstrates that these patients exhibit modifications of brain perfusion not found in healthy subjects and reinforces the idea that fibromyalgia is a 'real disease/disorder.'"

Fibromyalgia is a chronic disorder characterized by widespread muscle pain and fatigue. It affects 2%-4% of people, mostly women. It has been called the "invisible syndrome" because it can't be diagnosed based on a lab test or X-ray." (WebMD 2008)

My Exacerbations & Experiences

What is it like to have Multiple Sclerosis and Fibromyalgia (in other words, how will it affect a person physically)?

When I think of topics to add to this writing, I try to remember what things I wanted information on when I first got my MS diagnosis. Even though every patient is different, and even though medications affect different patients in different ways, I thought that reading about what I go through may be helpful. I apologize to you in advance if it is not and I urge you to consult with a physician if you need medical advice (because I am a patient and not a medical professional).

By the way, I am aware of the repetition of/varied forms of the adjective "different" in the previous paragraph and elsewhere in this book. It is no wonder to me that there is no cure for MS yet when there is so much variety with it (patient-to-patient, day-to-day).

I think I am going to try the "short list" first. I want to go over the exacerbations (also called attacks and flare-ups or flares) that I have had and that were "visible" to me. It is possible to have an

MS attack without knowing it's happening. I will start with my first health issues that I believe led and/or contributed to the first MS Attack that I had in 94.

From the moment I was born and during my early childhood I was sick practically all the time. I also had very bad allergies that led me to getting shots at a hospital about two times a week. This was while I was still very young (it would have been prior to me being in the sixth grade.) I have spoken to others with "Invisible Disabilities" and we have discovered that quite a large number of us had similar problems with regards to allergies and medications during our childhoods. Not every single one, but many.

Skipping on to my "young adult" years: It was the middle of 1994 and I was dating someone who didn't appear (at the time, to me) to care about me the way I cared about him. Adam and I had been together for almost two years and after all that time we still were only seeing each other on the weekends. We would meet at a dance club on Saturday nights and would go back to where he lived in the evenings afterward. He was approximately forty minutes away by car and about 90 minutes by train.

It's Not as Bad as it Sounds

I started getting Urinary Tract Infections (UTIs) while I was dating Adam. I won't go into a lot of detail about that here as I cover it under the section, How Did this Start and Where Did Things Go? but I will say that I started getting them regularly in a short period of time. After a while, I was getting them monthly. I joined a yearlong study involving drinking Cranberry juice to see if it helped (it did.) The reason behind the UTIs remained a mystery until I found out about having MS.

Later in my relationship with Adam, I started having trouble breathing. I was wheezing when I inhaled and at times it felt like the oxygen wasn't going into my lungs. I was with Adam and had to take an early train to get to the hospital (Adam had a truck but he made me take the train). I had to get to the ER on my own. I didn't feel that Adam was being the most caring and supportive boyfriend he could have been, but I believe he had to get to work that day. I took the train into the city and went to the Hospital. I got to the Emergency Room (ER) and was put on an oxygen tank almost immediately. I was eventually given an inhaler and told I had bronchitis and that it would go chronic if I didn't quit smoking cigarettes.

This seemed (at the time) like an isolated incident but I wonder if it contributed to what happened next. A few months after this happened I started having my first bout of "optic neuritis". I did not know that is what I had because I had never had any eye problems before (I had perfect vision at this point) and I had no idea that I had Multiple Sclerosis. As I said in another section (under My MS & Fibro Journey), I didn't know what was wrong. I thought I had an odd form of pinkeye or something. I went to the hospital and found out I had something far more serious, but nobody appeared to know exactly what was wrong.

My pupils were two different sizes and when I looked diagonally at anything it doubled and or tripled in my vision. I was told I might have a brain tumor. Apparently our attacks can easily be mistaken for other things (I also found out I could have been given tests to make sure I wasn't a "stroke victim"). I didn't get a diagnosis after all this. I was told I might have MS or Lupus but nobody knew precisely what was wrong. I mentally blew it off completely. Looking back I'm kind of glad I did this. It was almost a full year before I had health problems again and that year of not thinking I had medical problems was a pretty good year. It was easier to put this out of my mind because I also did not feel that I had anyone I could confide in about it. I certainly didn't feel I could tell my boyfriend Adam what was happening.

Approximately a year later (towards the end of 1994) I had another odd vision problem. The hardest part about this "eye problem" was that I couldn't come up with a way to describe what was happening. Thankfully, I was working at a place that had healthcare benefits and I was working in a medical area. It turned out this was another "bout" of optic neuritis. I went to see my PCP who sent me to a Neuro-Ophthalmologist (an eye doctor who specializes in people with Neurological disorders). I was given a visual field test that showed I had a blind spot in the same spot in both eyes. I was then sent to have my second MRI and a "visual evoked potential" exam after my doctor told me he suspected MS based off of the MRI results. I was assigned to a Neurologist.

Unfortunately, the Neurologist my PCP referred me to did not specialize in working with people who had Multiple Sclerosis. He was definitely not a "people person" and he also wasn't particularly helpful or responsive at all. All he did was confirm the diagnosis, unnecessarily scare my mother and me, and then become impossible to reach; he would not even return phone calls or emails.

As little as I knew about my condition, I knew I needed a different Neurologist. While my mom was with me I had asked this Neurologist to give me an example of what an attack was like. He used a very bad example (a "worst case scenario") that got my mother and me extremely upset. He told me he had a woman who came in saying her left arm was "tingling". He then told me her entire left side wound up paralyzed a week later.

How are we, as patients, expected to react to being told something like this? As I have mentioned in the section My MS and Fibro "Journey", this was an incredibly bad example he used to describe an MS attack. After this, my mother would call me almost daily to make sure I was OK. If my allergies started acting up, she and I would BOTH panic about what was going to happen to me.

It took me a long time to get over what this
Neurologist had told us. It took my mother twice as
long - she had to meet another Neurologist who was
able to reassure her. She had a VERY hard time
coming to terms with the fact that I had this
"MonSter" but after hearing the horrible example
the first Neurologist gave us of an MS attack,
coming to terms with knowing her daughter had it
was much harder than it should have been.

Thankfully, I found a very good Neurologist next
(an MS Specialist). This was in part from working
in a medical area but it was also from speaking
with my local chapter of the National Multiple

Sclerosis Society (NMSS). The MS Neurologist I went to was in the same hospital as the Neuro who diagnosed me, and when our appointment came to a close he told me I could come to him or go back to the first Neurologist I saw for my next appointment. When I told him the example the first Neurologist had given me, my new Neurologist got a bit upset and told me it was crazy to give an example like that to someone who "obviously has such a mild case of this condition" and that something like this was too far fetched to offer as an example of what I should expect to face. This new MS specialist remained my Neurologist for a few years. I absolutely loved having him as my doctor. Unfortunately, he became extremely popular (he was also very involved in doing research on MS) and was, therefore, very hard to find/see so I wound up eventually changing doctors and hospitals.

Montel Williams was diagnosed with MS in 1999 and he had a Neurologist at Brigham and Women's' Hospital (BWH). With a little bit of research on the web and, after discussing him with people I worked with in the medical area, I found out that he had given some money to Brigham and Women's Hospital (which helped them open an MS Center) and that he had an MS Specialist there. I decided to follow his progress since he looked like he was doing well to me. I wanted to know his "secrets" if he had any.

What impressed me about him most was how he used exercise to help with his day-to-day MS symptoms. When I got myself back into a gym "routine" I remember telling one of the faculty members I worked for what I was doing. He then asked me if I could bench press the weight level that Montel could. I laughed, said "no" and then told him I might not be strong enough to do it yet but that my goal was to become that strong. I still have arms that aren't as strong as they should be but I am glad I decided to follow the path of exercise and healthy eating that I had discovered when researching Montel.

The "healthful living" may not have cured me but it eventually made me feel much better both physically and psychologically. Thankfully, I not only decided to follow in Montel's footsteps as far as healthful living is concerned, but I also eventually switched to his hospital after my Neurologist became so hard to stay in touch with. I am getting a little bit ahead of myself here so I am now going to move on to the next attack I had.

About a year after the second bout of optic neuritis, I had another (at the time) difficult to describe attack. It happened on a bus-ride to work. I got off the bus and suddenly felt like I was being pulled, as if by magnetic force, to the left. I then became extremely dizzy. I had to let my boss know what was going on and then I had to go home. The dizziness/vertigo was horrible – I had a very hard time walking because of it. This went on for a few days and I finally went to my primary care physician (PCP). Unfortunately, my PCP was another doctor I was not too happy about. I chose him because he was my mother and stepfather's doctor and I respected their opinion of him. They both felt he was a very good doctor (and he was, to them). He was not a good doctor to my husband, and me however.

While this attack was going on, I should have gone to see my Neurologist or at least tried to contact him first. However, I thought my insurance company required a referral from my primary care doctor to see another specialist. Unfortunately my PCP continued to ignore that there was anything physically wrong with me, even after I was diagnosed with Multiple Sclerosis. He once told my mother he thought I was "extremely proactive" about my healthcare which I took as a very diplomatic way of calling me a hypochondriac. When I told him what was going on with the dizziness and the vomiting it was causing he told me he was sure I was having an inner ear infection.

I was also asked if there was any possibility I could be with child and experiencing morning sickness. I was tested for this and was able to verify that I was not. At some point I had a doctor tell me I probably could no longer get pregnant. I honestly wish I could remember who it was who told me this. Years later, right before I had a supracervical hysterectomy to remove fibroids, I got my period for the fist time in years. This leads me to believe that I may have been able to get pregnant after all. I am very, very fortunate that I never did.

My PCP refused to do anything beyond this point and he also would not give me a referral to see my Neurologist. I eventually decided to take matters into my own hands and I made an appointment to see him (my Neuro) on my own. Thankfully he took what I was going through very seriously. He told me I was having a classic MS attack and he told me this by being very diplomatic (in other words, he did not badmouth my PCP but did say he could not understand why the doctor refused to consider that I was having an exacerbation when I was exhibiting "classic MS symptoms"). I was given Antivert to control the dizzy feeling. The phrase 'the room is spinning" is not one I can take lightly, particularly not after having gone through this experience. It was awful. When the room is spinning and all you are doing is lying on your bed trying to fall asleep it is very hard to keep fighting to persevere. Even though the temptation to give up can be very strong at times it is more than worth pushing onward, in my opinion.

For my next attack the dizziness came back with a vengeance and I couldn't hold anything down (liquid or solid). I was now a patient at Brigham and Women's Hospital with another good MS Neurologist. I was put on an IV steroid treatment for the flare-up. Unfortunately, it didn't help me much at all. Bear in mind that I know of many other MS patients who have benefited from the steroid treatments but as I have stated before, different medications work differently for different people.

The only thing(s) that helped with the nausea were the Meclizine pills and time. Additionally, I have since learned that drinking water has the potential to make things much worse with regards to nausea. This was something I did not know at the time of this attack, unfortunately. One thing I have learned since is that drinking ginger ale and/or ginger tea with honey would have been a much better choice. This particular flare lasted just under two weeks.

Approximately one year later, I had the worst attack I have ever had (before or since). My left arm went numb and this brought back the memory of what my first Neurologist told me about the patient who wound up temporarily paralyzed on one side. One major problem with a disease like MS is not knowing what is going to happen next. Despite everything I had been told about having such a "mild case" of MS, I couldn't help but wonder where the numbness in my arm and hand would lead. Thankfully the numbness remained localized in my left arm but this was still a fairly major problem for me because I am left-handed so I was unable to write.

As with every attack I have had, I had several left over side effects/symptoms from this one. I had (and continue to have) tingling and a lack of sensation in both of my hands. I also started having some significant pain problems. I thought the pain was just from the MS, initially. It took me a few years (along with getting burned out of my home, being laid off a year later, and then losing a very close family member a few years after that) to find out I also had Fibromyalgia. What the MS and the medications did to me along with all of the stressors may have been contributing factors to me developing the Fibro "syndrome". However, I do not know that I will ever be certain what caused it or precisely when it developed.

Despite all of the physical problems having these conditions can cause, the biggest challenge with having an invisible disability is often the way others view and/or treat us. The way people act towards people with invisible disabilities is a never-ending battle (of sorts). It is frustrating and feels unfair that those of us who have these health problems have to constantly prove that something is wrong. I understand that, many times when we have to prove ourselves to others, it is because they do not understand. This does not change how hard it is on us (the patients) when we are not believed.

I just want to state as a side note to all friends, family members and loved ones of people who have these "invisible" illnesses (if you are reading this book you may not need this but perhaps you can share it with anyone who might): whether you can see something is wrong with us or not is not what matters. What is relevant is that you are someone we should be able to depend on and having you call us a liar, or lazy, or any of the other horrible things that you may want to label us is incredibly unfair and hurtful. How would you feel if someone did something like that to you? Is it that hard for you to attempt to empathize with us? It should not be. Just because you cannot see what is happening does not mean it is not. If you are married to someone with an invisible illness please do not forget the vow you made to love your partner "in sickness and in health." You made a commitment and you should stand by it.

There are support groups for caregivers to people with these medical conditions. I know that the demands of being a caregiver can be overwhelming and I am not trying to heap a bunch of blame on you. However, please understand that I have heard horror stories about parents, siblings, and/or partners who were abusive and/or unwilling to try to learn what they were doing (or not doing) wrong. I know you did not ask to be "saddled" with someone with a disability, but we did not ask to be sick either.

Here is a link to a video by Kristie Salerno Kent about living with MS. This is, in my opinion, helpful for explaining what having MS feels like. I have shared it with many others. In my opinion it is wonderful:

http://tinyurl.com/at2awf

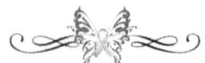

Our Pasts – Can They Lead to Future Health Problems?

I am going to begin a new "section" here but I have a feeling this is going to branch out into the rest of what I write. I find from talking to other MS and Fibro patients that a LOT of us have had horrible experiences growing up that either followed or "found" us in adulthood. I have to wonder if our immune systems had to go into overtime to help us get through some of the ordeals we went through.

My childhood was not the worst but it was definitely not fun either. You couldn't pay me enough money to make me choose to go back in time. I was a picked on/bullied child in school all the way up to my last year in high school. I was also a runaway; I ran away twice and I never returned after my second try. College was a fun experience the first time around but I didn't get out of it what I should have. I (much) later received my degree in 2012.

Bear in mind that my intent was not to get hung up on things having to do with my parents because this book was not originally intended to just be an autobiography. This chapter will read like one, however. I was surprised at how much time I spent going on about my father here. I apologize for how long this is but I must admit that writing it led me to realize things about myself and my upbringing that I was not fully aware of – I suppose one might say that writing this was very cathartic.

Despite not wanting to only focus on my own "life story", I do want to go over some problems that I had during my childhood and beyond as I feel these things all could have contributed to the Multiple Sclerosis manifesting in me. I also have gone into as much detail as I have here to share my story with you and to invite you to share back if you wish.

I'm always hearing about how stress can be physically bad for us and I definitely believe it's true. I also have spoken with many others who have MS (and/or other invisible disabilities such as Fibro, Lupus, Spina Bifida, etc.) about this and many have told me some serious "school of hard knocks" stories. I am astounded at the horrible things my close friends in the disabled community have told me they went and/or go through either growing up and/or with their family, friends and colleagues currently.

I think a lot of us have more in common than we realize. I know that science has found that, the further away a person lives from the equator, the more likely they are to develop MS. However, I have to wonder if the stressful backgrounds we come from are contributing factors. I truly think they are.

Like almost everyone else I know and/or grew up with, I am a child of divorce. I spent the first year of my parents' break-up living with my mother. Things were really bitter between my mom and dad at this point. I wound up going to live with my father after the first year. I stayed with him until I was sixteen years old. I hope this section will illustrate some of the hardships I have had in an effort to show others that they are not alone in much of what they have had to face.

Even though I was very young when my parents split up (I was just getting into the fifth grade of school. I believe I was eight), I remember having an insight into things I had many counselors speak to me about. I remember knowing that the break-up was not my fault. I also remember understanding that it was wrong for one parent to demonize the other to their child and therefore realized my father was wrong in constantly badmouthing my mother to me. Despite getting this, I never told anyone he was doing it. He did this the first year (after the breakup) when I lived with her and he continued to do it the entire time I lived with him.

Every weekend I would fly between New York and Massachusetts to visit him and he would show me a tin can he was filling up with money. He would tell me the money would be mine if I ever came to live with him (this tin can will be brought up again later in this section).

My father did not appear to know that badmouthing an ex-spouse to your child immediately after a breakup was a bad thing to do. I recall being proud of myself in that I thought I was mature and/or clever enough to understand that what he was doing was wrong. I was able to make up conversations I had with my mother to please him. Whenever my mom and I would get together he would "prep" me by giving me things to say to her. When I was back with him he would then ask me to report back on her responses to them as well as give me "ideas" of things to say the next time I saw her. This went on for many years after I ended up living with him.

It never dawned on me that I should have asked for help from an adult or at least informed one of what was going on. Then again, there were no adult figures I felt I could approach in the first place. I did once tell a so-called friend what my dad was doing and, when I was done, she told me she thought I was crazy. To this day I cannot understand why that was her reaction to everything I told her. I guess she just could not deal with the reality of it. Her somewhat callous response was not helpful to me at all. She just made me feel more alone and isolated than I did before. I had not told anyone else what was going on and this was the response I got from someone who I thought was a close friend. Now I felt certain that there was nobody I could tell.

Regardless of all of this, I couldn't picture myself as a "victim" of emotional/verbal abuse. I didn't realize I was a victim until I lived with him for about four more years. As intelligent as I thought I was, I was not smart enough to see that he would never stop putting my mother down even after I went to live with him. He didn't stop talking badly about her until very recently and I think he stopped because he finally realized how upset and angry it made me the last time he did it.

He picked a very bad time to do it too – I had just called him to tell him my stepfather Martin (who I was very close to) had passed away and he told me he was sorry I was sad but that my mother was "dead to him". I was not expecting him to be completely supportive about my stepfather. I realized that Martin had been married to my father's ex-wife, but my mother and father had been divorced for over 25 years at this point. I was extremely sad and hoping for a father figure to speak with. I was calling my dad to cry and make sure he knew I loved him because another father figure in my life had just died. Having him say my mother was "dead to him" at this point in my life was just too much for me to take; I hung up on him.

He has since apologized to me for that and for his anger at women in general. He seemed to finally get how much it was dividing us. Now that I have "fast forwarded" too much here I am going to get us back to the point when I was a child living with my dad after my mom left him. I apologize for the abrupt time "jumps".

When I was living with my father, I did not truly understand that he was putting me in a position I shouldn't have been in every time he would make up nasty things for me to say to my mother and/or when he would tell me bad things about her. My mom recently told me that she felt really bad about the way the breakup went for him and that she didn't feel he did anything horrible to her. She said the only thing she felt any anger towards him over was what he put me through. She said (and she was correct) that he should NEVER have "dumped all of that" on me.

It's Not as Bad as it Sounds

I was only eight years old and this man was telling me my mother cheated on him as well as telling me with whom. He tried to make me feel like her leaving was partly because of me; he always said she left us both even though she took me with her. I also remember trying to get him to get a girlfriend. He told me that he tried dating someone and she didn't like that he had a daughter so he gave up and never tried to meet anyone again (that I am aware of). So, on top of making me feel partially to blame for the divorce, he made me feel responsible for keeping him single. While I realize my father never deliberately did any of this to hurt me, it was still a very hard thing to live through/with.

I apologize in advance for the racial slur I am going to use in this next paragraph: To add insult to injury, he and I went and stayed with some friends of his in Florida. His good friend's wife called my mother a "good for nothing Kike" right in front of me and I felt powerless to say anything back to her. She was German; I do not point this out this to be racist but it is pertinent to this section. I was very upset to hear her speak about my mother the way she did. At the time I believe I was ten years old and was starting to see the disadvantaged situation I was in. It really shocked me to hear a German woman use such racist language against a woman with a Jewish heritage. I had learned a little bit about the Holocaust in school and I remember thinking she had a lot of nerve to be badmouthing anyone Jewish, let alone my mother. This was not the only time she did this. In order to avoid having my father get angry with me I felt I had to pretend to agree with all of the horrible things she said.

Whenever we would see them this sort of talk would happen. Whenever it did I had to just sit and keep my mouth shut even though I had some choice words that I wanted to scream at her along the lines of "who do you think you are?" for starters. It wouldn't have been pretty and would have probably accomplished nothing except to get me into a LOT of trouble. It didn't help that this woman (and her daughter) were both very racist; not just against Jews but against every "minority" group out there. Their bigotry was inconceivable to me. This sort of racism still deeply offends me and probably always will.

Another thing my mother brought up to me recently was how surprised she was that I wanted to live with my father in the first place. Looking back on my life now, I can certainly understand her surprise. I was afraid of him. He was always so angry. A very early memory I have of him was when I was in kindergarten. I remember him spanking me and yelling that he wouldn't stop hitting me until I stopped crying. I do not know how long this lasted. I do remember that he did not stop until my mother came home, saw what he was doing, and made him stop. I do not remember what I did to "earn" the spanking. However, I do not understand how anyone could think that hitting a young child while screaming they would stop as soon as the kid stopped crying could be effective. It did not work for me; the spankings got harder as his anger grew more intense. I was probably crying more out of fear than anything else at this point. I think he was just angry and getting himself worked up as he was spanking me. In my opinion this was abuse, not discipline.

Moving on through childhood: as I have written before, I was a bullied child. This started in the first grade and didn't stop until I entered my senior year of high school. I went to Catholic school from the sixth until the eleventh grade. My senior year of high school was at a public school in the Bronx, New York. I probably got picked on because when I was growing up I had absolutely no sense of humor. I was also horrible at anything and everything gym related and I am certain the MS had something to do with that. I had a bad tremor and my equilibrium was never normal. I do not think that knowing I had MS would have prevented the other children from picking on me, however. Unfortunately bullies are just cruel. A particularly bad gym memory I have is of a dodge ball game. I do not remember what grade I was in but I do remember my own team cheering when I got hit and had to go to the bleachers. It was humiliating.

After my parents broke up and while I was living with my mother I went from school to after-school camp. I was bullied in camp too. I remember reading about "latchkey kids" (i.e., children who went to an empty home after school due to their parents being away at work) and wishing my mom would let me be one. I thought that I would be happier at home by myself rather than being in camp with a bunch of children (and in one case a camp counselor who told me she didn't like me and asked me to stay away from her – I was nine at the time) who couldn't stand me.

So school and after-school camp (and summer camp) were nightmares for me. In a baseball-like game at camp there was another child who almost seriously injured me. She threw a ball at my head and it missed me by centimeters. It took a fairly large piece out of the tree it hit right next to me though. As this went on I continued to get sick fairly frequently. I didn't mind however - being sick kept me from having to go to school.

When I was in the fifth grade a male student came up to me and grabbed, squeezed and twisted my breasts right in front of our professor. She (the teacher) watched this happen and did absolutely nothing about it. I later found out that my mother did not care for her. Apparently at a parent-teacher meeting she met her and was told that she "hated children." Obviously being a fifth-grade teacher was a very bad career choice for her. Despite her negative feeling towards kids she should have done something about the boy who accosted me right in front of her. There were other students who physically came after me. I also had one who lived right near me and he used to chase me on his bike every day on the way home from camp.

Looking back I think I was hoping for school to be better if I got to move in with my father. I don't know why I thought that would happen and I don't know why I was so miserable living with my mother. I think the fact that we were living in poverty had a lot to do with it, despite the fact that she managed to hide it from me very well at the time. In addition, as smart as I thought I was as to what my father was doing when he talked negatively about my mother, I believe he successfully poisoned my mind against her. I blamed her for all the horrible things I went through at school. I blamed her for everything.

It's Not as Bad as it Sounds

I believe it is Pink who has a song about communicating to her 16-year-old self. I wish I could go back in time and speak to the me that was just getting through my parents splitting up so I could tell myself that there was no shame in getting an adult involved in what I was going through.

I was wrong in thinking about school getting better when I went to go live with my father. It stayed bad and I remained a "bullied child" until I ran away from home. I don't know why children are so mean to each other. I think part of it is the feeling of being powerless and/or the loss of independence combined with peer pressure and potential family problems that is hidden from others. I'm sure that even some of the most popular kids have a lot of emotional issues that they have to deal with. Add to this the fact that when one child is bullied and/or picked on by the majority (regardless of the reason), the "majority rules." How can this sort of thing not lead to mean-spirited interactions?

When I lived with my father he wanted me to go to Catholic school. He wanted to distance me from my mother as much as he possibly could. My mother is an artist and, as a result of his anger towards her, any interest I exhibited towards the arts made him angry and resentful. He took his anger out on me by yelling at me and forbidding me to have anything to do with being creative.

This was a problem for me as I have always had an interest in drawing, painting and creative writing. He pretty much destroyed my chances at doing anything "artsy" while I lived with him. I had a lot of illustrations and writings that I did while growing up that I wound up throwing away. I would love to get all or even some of that artwork back but it is all gone.

On top of constantly yelling at me, he would often act very unhappy and sad and would sometimes guilt me into thinking I was causing him to feel unwell because I was acting so much like my mother. I do not think he did this intentionally though. I think he was so hurt by the divorce (his second) that it really did get to him and manifest itself physically. Unfortunately, he often made me feel like I was the reason behind his sadness.

I'm fortunate that he never physically abused me but I remember wishing he would do that instead of psychologically/verbally abusing me. I think I wanted him to hit me and to leave bruises so I could prove what he was doing. Everyone who met my father thought he was wonderful and nobody was able to see what he was doing to me.

It's Not as Bad as it Sounds

Another thing I should note about my father is how much older he is than my mother (I believe they are about twenty years apart in age). He is very old fashioned and, as a result of being born deaf and not learning his native tongue correctly (and therefore not learning English properly), he had many communication problems.

When I was fifteen I remember hanging out with some friends near where we lived and having him come by and scream at me in front of them for not wearing a brassiere. I was very top heavy and he told me I looked like a prostitute when I didn't wear a bra. My friends (females and males) appeared to be uncomfortable and a little embarrassed that he would say that to me in front of them. I was horrified. I always had a bit of a complex about my breasts (I had reduction surgery in 1998) but having him do this certainly did not help.

I had so many bad experiences while I was living with him that I began to go a little out of my mind. I had it pointed out to me by a friend's mother that she saw me sitting on a bench staring off into space and that I didn't react when she tried to get my attention. I also had a few experiences where I would realize I had been crying without knowing it. I felt that there was absolutely no way out. I started hurting myself. I think I just wanted someone to notice me at first but I got desperate when I couldn't get the attention I was seeking. I then made the mistake of meeting with a counselor at my school (she was a nun) and telling her I didn't want to live anymore. Her "helpful response" was to tell me I would burn in hell if I killed myself. She offered me no useful advice whatsoever.

As I lived with my father and as I came to understand how miserable I was and would continue to be, I asked him to send me to a therapist. He became angry and yelled that no child of his was crazy. He refused continuously to send me in for counseling. I reached my "breaking point" towards the end of my junior year of high school. After a (thankfully) unsuccessful attempt at suicide, I knew I needed to see someone so I could tell him/her what I was going through. Since my dad was still so mad at my mom for leaving him I decided to try to use his anger to my advantage. I asked to meet with a therapist and told him it had to do with my mother. I was right – as soon as he thought I needed to see someone over being upset about her he sent me right away.

I don't think this therapist was expecting our meeting to go the way it did. I told her everything. When we were done, she asked to speak with my father alone in her office. I sat out in the waiting area for what felt like an incredibly long time.

It's Not as Bad as it Sounds

When they were done meeting, she walked out of her office with him and called me back in to speak with her in private. I thought I was going to get yelled at.

Instead of yelling at me or giving me useless advice, she asked me if there were any adult figures I knew who I could live with. She told me she did not usually advise people the way she was about to advise me, but that she thought I would be much better off living with someone else if that was an option. I took this as my (eventual) queue to leave. My first time running away wasn't very successful. I ran away and went to live with a friend. I lived with her and her mother for a week and then my father found me and forced me to come back home.

A short time after this I ran away again. This time the friend who I went to live with a few weeks prior wanted to come with me. She told me her biological father, who lived in Connecticut, had agreed to take us in. We went to Penn Station in New York City to get on a train to go out there. A friend of hers' (the girl I ran away with) called the cops and gave them our descriptions. He told them we were prostitutes and we wound up getting handcuffed and brought in for questioning.

It's Not as Bad as it Sounds

At the time I was very upset by this but it turned out to all be for the best. Mary's father had never agreed to let us come live with him (I don't even know if she ever really got in touch with him). Another thing I didn't know was that Mary planned on us both killing ourselves if things didn't "work out" with our attempt at running away. When the cops brought us in for questioning they put us in separate rooms. Mary didn't have any paperwork with her so she was questioned for a long time; longer when the cops found the pills she was planning on us using to poison ourselves with if things didn't go our way. I had all of my paperwork with me (school ID, birth certificate, any other paperwork I could find and a box filled with change and some dollar bills).

Mary finally got put on the phone with her mother and my father was at her mom's house. When Mary was done speaking to her mother, I got put on the phone with my dad. The first thing he asked me was if I stole the money he kept in the tin can in his dresser. I answered that yes I had taken the money but that I didn't consider it theft because he had told me growing up that I could have it if and when I came to live with him. When I told him this he got quiet for a few moments and then told me I was no longer his daughter and hung up on me.

It's Not as Bad as it Sounds

For the first time I was finally free but I was also terrified since I had no idea what was going to happen next. I didn't know where I was going to go and I certainly didn't expect Mary's mom to offer to let me stay with them since I had been about to run away from home with her daughter. Fortunately for me my mother's brother, who also lived in New York City, offered to let me stay with him and his wife.

I am going to skip ahead some years here because, even though I know it is too late to state this, I don't want to get completely "bogged down" in my own life story outside of the "invisible disabilities" that I have. I do, however, want to cover other things that led up to the MS diagnosis. My senior year of high school was a big improvement for me now that I was no longer living with my father and no longer in Catholic school. I had to work and do a lot of household chores to help my Uncle and his wife but I was very happy compared to the way I was prior to running away. My life got much better when I left to go to College.

I went to school full time for two years as a creative writing major. I didn't really take college as seriously as I should have and I dropped out after my second year because I thought I could finish it anytime I wished. I was very much mistaken about that. I was too young and foolish to realize how much life could and eventually would get in the way.

After I dropped out of the State University of New York (SUNY) that I had been attending, I moved to Massachusetts back to where my mother had gone to when she left my dad. I began working right away and I enjoyed making money and being able to afford my own place to live so much that I forgot about school for a long time. I didn't start going back until I got a job somewhere that offered tuition assistance as an employee benefit. I tried going back part time and I took a few classes here and there, but finishing up and getting my degree felt like an impossibly long "project." I didn't think

I would ever be able to graduate and get a College degree.

In 1994 I got a job at a very well known University in Massachusetts. While I was working there I got diagnosed with MS. I was very fortunate in that I had a job with benefits at this point in my life. I also met my husband while I worked at the University. I worked there for eleven years and over ten months before I was laid off.

A year before getting laid off, my husband and I got burned out of our home thanks to an over fifty-year old water heater in the basement of the building.

It's Not as Bad as it Sounds

We lost everything we had. I am very thankful that, years before the fire, I followed my mother's advice and got apartment renters' insurance.

We had friends that we stayed with for a few weeks after the fire but being homeless for a little over a month was incredibly stressful, to say the least. It didn't dawn on me how lucky we were to have survived until months after the fire destroyed our building. Looking back, I think I might have been laid off a little bit sooner had it not been for being burned out. A while after I was told I had been laid off I found out that others I worked with had known and/or suspected that my being let go was "in the cards" almost a year prior to it happening.

Yvonne Decelis

After I was laid off, I wound up working several different jobs and found myself struggling just to make ends meet. I could not find a job like the one I had been laid off from because everyone was looking for someone with a Bachelors degree. I had a few of the worst jobs I have ever had during this time.

During this period in my life I had some really bad experiences with supervisors/bosses. In one position I reported to a woman half my age who yelled at me on my first day. I probably should have anticipated this – I was the "second choice" for this job as their original hire quit after working there for one month. Even though I met with someone to discuss the problems I was having with my boss (while I still worked at this company), nobody appeared to understand that she was the problem with keeping the job filled. To this day they can't seem to keep anyone in this position. I recently looked at an online job board and I found a listing for it.

The fire and the layoff were major stressors, to say the least. These combined with having to work at low-paying jobs that I couldn't stand likely made my health problems worse. Unfortunately after I was laid off my former employer made finding a career particularly hard for me. I believe that someone in their Human Resources (HR) department disclosed about my illness to at least two potential employers. I know of many others (some who work there and some who do not) that believed the same thing. Either they told potential employers I had MS or told them I had "mental issues." As a result of this, I found it impossible to find a decent job. So you do not think I am writing this out of resentment, let me give two examples that led me to this belief. I was offered a job by one employer and, as agreed, I came back to discuss a start date with them. I was informed that the job offer had been revoked because my prior employer had been contacted and they had stated that they felt the job would be too stressful for me. They had told this employer that I should only be offered something part time "for my own sake".

Another position I was interviewed for was denied after I was called in for four meetings for it. During my fourth meeting I was informed that I was the strongest candidate for the job. I was then told I would be asked to come in one more time before being offered the position. I waited almost two and a half weeks and then called and left a message for the faculty member who had been interviewing me. About a week after I left the message, she emailed me to let me know she was "surprised and disappointed" I had not been contacted by her HR department to be told I was no longer being considered as a candidate. I was given no reason as to why my candidacy had been removed. All I know is that the faculty member went from being very friendly while she was conducting the interviews to being distant and evasive in her final message to me. I replied to tell her that, while I was disappointed that I was no longer in contention for it, I wanted to wish her the best of luck with whomever she chose to fill the position. I never heard from her again.

My former employer had no reason to give me a bad reference, by the way. My employee record at their location had nothing in it but accolades. I even won a Customer Service award that I had to accept my last week there. There was no reason for me to have lost jobs because of them – they must have reported something they were not supposed to.

Since I suspected my former employer of disclosing about my illness, I hired a lawyer who agreed to work with me on a contingency basis. However, despite her assurances to the contrary, we did not have a chance. We went to the Massachusetts Commission Against Discrimination (MCAD) and lost there.

I had gotten a letter before being laid off warning me that I was costing my employer over a thousand dollars a month because of all of the medical appointments I had for my MS. If I had had this letter at the MCAD trial we may have had a chance but it had been destroyed in the fire the year before.

The lawyer I hired then said we had a "really good case" that she was going to take to a higher court. Unfortunately, she (the lawyer) disappeared on me and I was so busy struggling to find work to make ends meet that I couldn't spend as much time hounding her as I should have. She got put on probation and she didn't tell me until almost a year after it happened. By the time I found out it was too late for me to do anything.

It's Not as Bad as it Sounds

Thankfully at this point I had applied for Social Security Disability insurance (SSDI) on my father's advice. Even though he had disowned me over the phone many years before, he and I were thankfully able to make peace with each other. We would never be as close as we once were again but were at least able to forge and maintain a friendly relationship by phone. I have my regrets about this and I always will.

Since I am about to move away from writing about my father (for this section) I feel I should mention a few other things: I have a half sister (on his side). As much as I complain about the things my father did to me, I must write that I feel they pale in comparison to what he did to her (or perhaps I should say what he didn't do since he abandoned her when she was very young). This is a seriously long story in itself and I don't want to go into her life tale although I really feel my father "did her wrong" in a big way.

I should say that I do not believe he meant to wrong her as badly as he did, however. I supposed one could say it was another argument for needing a "Parenting 101" instruction manual. Sadly there is no such guide. There should be, in my opinion. There should be a test you have to pass before you are given the right to have and raise children.

It's Not as Bad as it Sounds

Looking back on things as I write this, I realize that my getting diagnosed with MS has brought my father and me closer together. My grandmother began the process of patching things up between us after I ran away from home the second time but the MS completed it. Even though we live pretty far apart from each other I feel closer to him now than I have in a long time. He no longer badmouths my mother to me and sometimes asks me how she is doing.

Now to get back on track within this chapter: about three years after I applied for disability, and after getting rejected two or three times and then hiring a disability law group, I was approved for it. Since the University I had worked for before getting laid off paid me as well as they did, my disability pay was quite a bit higher than it was for many others that I knew who were on it. I certainly was not rich but I was at least able to afford the "basics" of life (rent and food).

I want to end this section on a positive note. I am doing this because it has been my experience that life is better (for me) when I "look at the bright side" of things. It is not always easy or possible to do but I do it whenever I am able. I recognize that, while I have gone through a lot of unpleasant things, I have also had some very significant strokes of good luck. I know things could have been much worse for me than they were. Having MS and Fibro is VERY unpleasant to say the least but I have been able to pull myself through and out of a lot of bad situations. I was finally able to go back to school and to graduate thanks to being on SSDI. I also became a fitness enthusiast since I had read and been told by a number of physicians that exercise was helpful in managing MS symptoms.

Despite being a bullied child in school, and despite all the problems I had in all of my gym classes, I loved working out at the gym(s) in the city of Boston and I became somewhat athletic. Ironically I was probably in better shape (in some ways) in my thirties than I was as a teenager. I still exercise whenever I am able to and I feel lousy when I don't make it to my gym. I also have a much healthier diet and I quit smoking in 2004.

Please remember that the subject of "background/life troubles" will probably come up again but I felt it was important enough to deserve its' own section. If you have any type of debilitating condition and you want to send me notes about things you went though, please do. I have found writing about this to be very therapeutic. I apologize for how long this section turned out to be but writing about it was surprisingly helpful to me and I'm hoping reading it helps you in some way too. I read recently that writing ones' life story can be the hardest thing a writer will ever do. I can understand why some may believe this to be the case but I have found that writing can sometimes help with lessening emotional pain, albeit gradually.

Yvonne Decelis

The "Art" Of Speaking Without Thinking

(AKA "foot in mouth")

I apologize in advance to anyone who is, in any way, affected by the condition "foot in mouth" or "hoof in mouth" disease. I am using the expression "foot in mouth" figuratively to discuss how so many people speak without thinking first (as well as a glimpse into the way this could potentially impact the person/people hearing it when this happen(s)).

It's Not as Bad as it Sounds

In this section I am going to (start to) go over the "foot in mouth" syndrome many people seem to develop when they come across people who have "invisible disabilities". This is not a complete list (far from it). Feel free to send me comments if you have gone through similar experiences. I have found that sharing it with others can have very therapeutic qualities.

When I was first diagnosed with MS I was a complete wreck. The chair of my office kept me busy the day I found out (so busy that I wound up having to stay and work late). I didn't mind this, however. I truly believe he was trying to take my mind off of what was going on since he saw how upset I was about it. If I had been married at the time I don't think I would have been happy about being kept busy. However, when I was diagnosed I was dating someone who wasn't the most helpful person in the world (emotionally) and I felt I didn't have anyone I could talk to.

To make matters worse, the Chair's secretary started treating me very badly. She was furious with me for staying at work the day I was diagnosed and she made sure I knew it. She also made sure I knew how upset she was with me for working late that day. According to her I had a "lot of nerve" staying in the office and bringing everyone "down with me." She also told me not to come back to work until I got over it. Seeing as how it took me close to two years to really "get over" finding out about the MS I am glad I ignored her incredibly unkind words.

It wasn't until about a year later that I found out her ex mother-in-law had MS and that, as soon as she found out I had it, she put me in the same "category" as her (ex) in-law. I also had some really thoughtless comments shared with me the week of my diagnosis. Bear in mind I was working in a hospital neighborhood at the time. I would have thought most people in the medical profession would know better but I was very much mistaken.

One person was trying to collect money on one of the main roads in the medical area that I worked at. As I was waiting for a bus to go home he walked up to me and told me that MS had "killed" his sister. He then asked for money and I said no, that I didn't appreciate his approach and that I wouldn't give him a penny. He acted horrified and said "I'm only trying to help people with MS!" to which I responded, "I JUST found out I have MS and you are in a Hospital neighborhood! Do you have any idea how awful it was to hear what you just said as a newly diagnosed MS patient?" He apologized and quickly walked away. I had a woman then walk over to me who said she was really proud of me for "putting him in his place". She was related to someone with MS and he had really upset her but she had just ignored him.

That same week I had someone point out to me that Richard Pryor had MS. I loved Richard Pryor and I knew he was sick but I had no idea he had MS. Being told that his illness was the same as what I had just been diagnosed with was not the most comforting thing to hear (at this point in time (1986) Richard Pryor was still alive but he was confined to a wheelchair).

People have a tendency to be a little thoughtless about things that do not affect them directly. I believe this is more often out of human nature than malice. There is also a "willful ignorance" and/or lack of empathy that many people with no serious health problems tend to have and/or exhibit towards us. This works both ways though. Sometimes people think they are being helpful and that they are showing empathy. That isn't always what is happening, however; statements like "everything happens for a reason", "just have faith", "I know just how you feel", etc. just make us (the people with the medical conditions) feel like we aren't understood and that we are being dismissed or, worse yet, blamed for our own medical problems.

It's Not as Bad as it Sounds

Throughout my writing I am sure I will have many more "foot in mouth" stories to tell you. To this day I still get some very thoughtless comments but since so much time has passed they don't hurt as much as they used to though they do sometimes make me angry and/or upset.

I'll never understand why people feel the need to blame patients for their medical problems. I know in some cases there is a fear that what we are going through could happen to them. Many times it is just ignorance of what we have to face. However the unwillingness to even try to empathize with and/or learn about our health issues is often incomprehensible to me.

I currently live in a building for elderly and disabled people and someone in my building saw me recently and told me I looked tired. I said I was and she said, "wow – if you're this tired now you'll never live to see 60!" I explained I had MS and "complete fatigue disability" but that didn't change her mind; she just repeated her statement. It made me a little angry but I just walked away. When people act like this their behavior can be poisonous to us. It usually is not worth our time (or our health) to allow ourselves to get worked up over it though. You can only teach people who are willing to learn, unfortunately.

It's Not as Bad as it Sounds

Bear in mind, however, that even people who are willing to learn many things aren't necessarily willing to learn about us. At a job interview for a Massachusetts (so-called prestigious) University, I disclosed about my illness and was then asked how long it would be before I was "completely useless". I wish I had known then that this was not legal and that I could have sued the man who asked me. He was a tenured Professor and he should have known better. Please know that I am not an overly litigious person but getting money from a lawsuit would have helped me avoid the horrible jobs I had after being laid off.

Yvonne Decelis

This type of thing (i.e., people in positions I would not have expected this type of behavior from) also goes the other way. I saw a doctor at one of the Massachusetts hospitals who refused to operate on my ankle when he found out I had MS. He got emotional on me, told me his grandmother had MS and then he said "MS is pain" (NOT true for all people with MS) and told me I should go on Oxycontin for the rest of my life. I'm glad I ignored him. I found another doctor and finally got the operation I was looking for. If I had taken the other doctor's advice I'm sure I'd be in much worse shape today (if I had been able to survive his medication suggestion).

It's Not as Bad as it Sounds

So in closing (for this section): it sucks and it is really unfair that we have to advocate for ourselves so much.

I am a member of a bunch of online support groups/blogs and one thing that never ceases to amaze me is the horrible behavior people in our shoes have to tolerate from their alleged friends, family members and or spouses / boyfriends / girlfriends. It's an outrage and it's a waste of our time and energy to have to tolerate these negative attitudes on top of what we have to deal with due to our own physical limitations. However, it is in our best interest to help each other out and to learn when we need to advocate for ourselves and to be pro-active about our health care.

There is one other thing I felt I needed to add to my "foot in mouth" section as an example of what I mean. I just remembered what my ex-boyfriend Adam said to me soon after I got my diagnosis of MS. A few weeks after I was diagnosed we went to a dance club that we used to go to weekly. We pulled into the parking lot and he turned to me and asked, "do you want to tell our friends or should I?" I stammered some response (don't remember exactly what it was) but I remember later telling him how upset this made me. I had finally been able to stop thinking about the fact that I had MS.

It's Not as Bad as it Sounds

This was my first night since being diagnosed where I felt I could let myself go out with the intention of having a good time and he dropped that on me in the parking lot right before we went in. I was very upset and angered by it and It ruined the entire evening for me.

He also once told me that he understood what I was going through with having MS because he had a disease too. I had absolutely no idea what he meant and, when I told him this, he said, "Oh - I'm an alcoholic." Once again I didn't immediately tell him how this made me feel. I told him the day we had our "final breakup" meeting. He dragged the break-up out for four weeks. He finally came to me with an art-pad full of notes as to why I shouldn't leave him. I told him how angry it had made me when he had compared his being an alcoholic to me having Multiple Sclerosis. He then tried to blame my anger on him on the MS. We definitely were on the road to a breakup with or without the diagnosis. After all, I should have felt I had someone to talk to when I was diagnosed but I certainly didn't feel that way about him. I told him that, while I was still very upset about the MS diagnosis, the breakup was something that had to happen and that MS was not in any way the reason for me wanting to end things between us. We had a long and somewhat uncomfortable conversation but thankfully it ended well (for me. I know he was very upset when things were over but I am also certain that he has found someone better suited to him).

MS is different from person to person. I've heard it (the disease) compared to snowflakes. Please know that every MS patient is different. I know of way too many people who think they can easily lump us into one group and/or category of people. Saying that people who have MS and/or Fibro (or any other invisible condition) is a "diverse group" cannot be over-emphasized.

A lot of people are completely unfamiliar with what Fibromyalgia is. I don't know if this is due to this "syndrome" not being as common as MS, but that is not a good reason to pretend it is a made up condition. Like MS, Fibro is more common in women than it is in men (according to research I have done, over ninety percent of Fibro cases are female. I believe MS is about three times more likely to occur in females than in males).

I recently had a friend tell me that she did not believe in it (knowing that I had it). Fibromyalgia is a very unpleasant condition to have. My own experience with it (regarding symptoms) is pain, increased fatigue, and cognitive troubles (often referred to as "Fibro fog"). Hearing someone say they think it is a "BS condition" is insulting. I am not sure how we are expected to respond to allegations like this. I remember (a long time ago) reading that people who have conditions like this tend to have emotional "imbalances". I also once read a comment on the web saying that we (MS patients) have "poor attitudes". With the types of things we have had to tolerate in addition to the physical suffering we endure on a constant basis, it amazes me that many of us are as kind and as positive as we are.

Please also know that if you are healthy and you hear someone with MS or Fibro say they are tired/in pain/experiencing "brain fog" (or similar types of complaints), you should not try to compare what they are feeling to yourself. I realize you may think you are being helpful but you probably are not. Just hear them out and nod politely if you can't think of anything to say.

We do not need (or want) you to tell us that you feel the same as we do. We need and/or want you to try to understand and believe what we are going through. If you try to compare what we are going through to something that happens to you it can come across as a "brush off." I realize that it can often be very hard to know what to say and that the temptation to compare what you feel to what we feel is strong. However, when I am feeling fatigued and someone healthy says something like "oh I get really sleepy too sometimes" I cannot help but feel a little frustrated (like what I just have said meant nothing). There is a big difference between feeling fatigued all the time no matter what and feeling very tired because you were up partying late the night before. Sometimes just saying "I'm sorry you feel that way" is enough. Sometimes we just need compassion. Just let us know you hear us and that you are there for us. Acknowledgment, compassion and understanding can all go a very long way for many of us.

The Online "Nay-Sayers"

(Why it may be a good idea to avoid the Internet and/or online resources when investigating health conditions.)

As I have written in many if not all other sections throughout this book I am a patient not a doctor. At this point in my life I have found a combination of medications that I feel work for me. I made the mistake of writing a post about this (in conjunction with an updated medical appointment with my Neurologist) in Facebook and had a couple of people write back that DMDs like Avonex (and all of the other Interferons/CRAB drugs) do not work and that combining them with LDN is a bad idea. They're most likely to be wrong (for me, it DOES work. It may not for all but it does for me). Either way, it was an exercise in futility and just led to a LOT of frustration (and tears) over absolutely nothing.

I suppose this just shows how little you can trust what you read online. To quote my neurologist on this subject: "...Just say that there are many studies that through the years showed the exact opposite results and they were not even sponsored by drug companies. The patients need to have hope that this illness can be controlled. Many studies support this hope. In the end, taking the medication is a personal decision for every patient. And even if it is proven beyond doubt that these drugs do not change the overall disability, or morbidity, the fact that the patients with MS are less likely to suffer exacerbations while taking therapies, which is an undisputed fact, is in and of itself, a wonderful thing. Going through exacerbations is best to be avoided, as it is very unpleasant, in a way that those without MS can't ever understand. The drugs work for some patients, do not work for other patients, and no two patients are the same. I would advise you to not waste your time writing a response. You can't change this person's mind, and it is not worth getting worked up about it in the process...."

She (my Neurologist) was right in my opinion.

I am adding this because I spend a LOT of time going over things that are Multiple Sclerosis-related. For anyone wanting to hear/read more about Fibromyalgia - I apologize. I have had MS for so much longer. The "world of Fibromyalgia" is still a little new to me. I am in a Sunset Tai Chi class (the teacher's name is Ramel Rones. He is WONDERFUL in my opinion) for people with Fibromyalgia. One of the people in my group is so negative all the time (she is truly upsetting to listen to). I try to cheer her up but I have had to back away and give up. Unfortunately, you can only do so much for other people.

Allowing too much negativity into our lives can be hazardous to our wellbeing. I feel very bad for this person but really hope, for her sake, that she can someday develop a more positive outlook. I have not really had too many online problems with Fibro because, to be honest, I still do most of my online research work (and reporting) on MS. I did, however, have one person tell me he thought I should not "compare MS and Fibro" when I told him the title of this book. I don't understand why he thought I was comparing them and I explained to him that I had both conditions. He then said he thought it was not worth going through "all sorts of unnecessary testing" to find out one had Fibro. I told him I didn't agree and that the tests for Fibro were not invasive or unnecessary at all.

One other thing I want to mention here is something my mother brought up in a comment in one of my writings about MS and Fibro. I read what she wrote and thought "hey – I could not have said this better myself" so I am just quoting what my mom wrote right here: "...Advice to the newly diagnosed: do NOT read listserv MS group messages. They are mostly from those with the worst cases and will only scare you to death. As Yvonne has said, each person with MS is different.

Also there have been great strides in medication so there are actually things that can help now that didn't exist 20 years ago. I was there when the doctors told her that she "might" have MS. They also said that if she had to get it, the timing was good because the first drug for MS, Betaseron, had just been approved. Before that there was nothing."

This is not just true about MS; I think you could probably say this about many medical conditions. If you search for something online chances are VERY good that you will find a lot of "worst case scenario" stories. If you just received a diagnosis or just found out someone you care about has something, you are probably not going to like what you find online. Please keep this in mind if you ever do decide to search for something on the Internet. Also know that, if you see any type of service announcement(s) in the media regarding a health condition where donations are being asked for, the worst possible cases are often shown in order to tug at the heartstrings of people who may have money to give.

Medications I Use (Rx, LDN)

Please remember as you read this that I am a patient, not a doctor. Also remember that MS is very different from person to person. I know I may sound like a "broken record" but so many people lump us all in the same category and that is not a good thing. I am going to go on to give information regarding some of the medications currently available for people with Multiple Sclerosis and will go into a little more detail about the medications I've taken myself. I am also leaving out all of the supplements I take (like fish oil tablets, magnesium, vitamins B and D, etc.) since they are all over the counter (OTC). I am not leaving these OTC meds out because they are not strong by the way; that is a fairly common misconception. Please do not ever make the assumption that, just because you can get something without a doctor's prescription, a medication (or food or drink) can't be harmful. I know people who have given themselves liver problems to the point of going into renal failure by taking OTC products, either due to taking too much of something and/or due to a bad drug interaction between the OTC medication and something else.

Bear in mind that this section (and others) may switch from current to past tense. That is because I am trying to update this to keep up with what is happening in my life but MS makes life very complicated, to say the least.

Finding out about having MS was a roller coaster ride. I found out I had it and I was very upset. Then I found out there was a medication available and the sadness started to dissipate. Then I found out the only thing available at the time of my diagnosis was an injectable medication (known to cause "flu like symptoms" and depression) that could later lead to serious liver damage.

It's Not as Bad as it Sounds

It's bad enough not knowing how you are going to feel in a day but finding out there were no oral "disease modifying drugs" (DMD) and that the only medications that were available were injectables with all sorts of known side effects certainly did not help. NOTE: Gilenya, Tecfidera, and Aubagio are the (as of now) newest oral disease modifying drugs (DMDs) to be approved for relapsing remitting MS. I will be switching to Tecfidera (AKA BG12) in a few weeks myself.

My first medication was one of the "CRAB" drugs *(Copaxone, Rebif, Avonex and Betaseron)*. I was only able to take this for a little under six months. It didn't help me, and the side effects made me feel a LOT worse. The first time I took it I woke up with horrible chills (this was on a day that was over one hundred degrees and humid in my area. It was like having an internal air conditioner that I couldn't turn down or off). The first one I tried was a subcutaneous injection; meaning under the skin as opposed to muscular or IV. I believe it was either an every-other-day or three times a week injection.

I had a bad attack while on this medication and I went off of it because not only did it make me feel horrible but it did not seem to be very effective (for me). Bear in mind that I know of many others who do benefit from this medication though – we all react differently so you cannot go by my own experiences with meds (and I know it is incredibly frustrating that we are all so different in this respect. It makes finding what will work much harder than it should be).

The next medication I went on to was Avonex, another CRAB drug. Avonex is a once a week intramuscular injection. I was very intimidated the first time I saw how big the needle was (twenty-three gage, one and a quarter inch length (Biogen 2013)). I called my Neurologist to tell him how shocked I was by the needle size. He told me that he couldn't understand why I would be so upset by this considering I had (at the time) numerous piercings. In my opinion this was not a good or helpful reply.

At least with piercings you have no "side effects" plus they are not something you have to do every week. I think many doctors also suffer from "foot in mouth syndrome" from time to time. It would definitely be nice if people would just think (and try to put themselves in our shoes) before they speak. A weekly intra-muscular injection is not the same thing as a tattoo or a piercing. Perhaps he thought his response was humorous but he was wrong if he did.

Like the first medication, Avonex also gave me horrible side effects that would make me sick for three to four days but it also appeared to be helpful for me in other ways. My reason for thinking it helped is that I haven't had an attack since 2000 (and I'm knocking-on-wood in the hope that I'm not jinxing myself by writing this) and because a few of the lesions that appeared on my MRIs diminished a bit since having been on it.

About three years ago I was told about a way to make the side effects far less potent (again – this works for me and several others but I can't promise that it will work for you). I spoke to a nurse in (approximately) early March of 2010 and, when I complained of how lousy the Avonex made me feel, she recommended I try eating fresh (i.e., unprocessed, uncanned, unheated) pineapple about an hour to thirty minutes before injecting because it has an enzyme in it (Bromelain) that helps lessen the side effects significantly. FYI: Bromelain is a natural anti-inflammatory. She reminded me that the pineapple had to be fresh in order for the enzyme to be present (but I did have one MS friend tell me she used canned and felt it still helped. Then again, another one of my "MSer" friends told me the exact opposite and swore that she would only use fresh pineapple from that point on). I found that the more pineapple I ate, the more it helped. Unfortunately I am not wild about pineapple aside from how well it worked with making the side effects tolerable. I loved it for that but not for the taste.

It's Not as Bad as it Sounds

My Neurologist also told me she had been telling her patients about this and that she was getting good feedback from them (for all of the Interferons, not just for Avonex). She also emphasized drinking lots of water the day of and after the shot. This was not a shocker to me since the "sickness" I felt after the shot felt a bit like a really bad hangover. An online friend of mine who has MS and who uses Rebif said the pineapple helped her tremendously.

I began making smoothies instead of eating the pineapple all by itself. The smoothies worked really well; I'm glad too. I got very tired of Pineapple (I have never been a fan but having to have it every week made me hate them after a few years). The only bad thing about this was that my body appeared to adapt to them. I recently tried to just eat pineapple and it didn't help at all so I now had to make myself a smoothie every time I did my shot. No matter how good the smoothie(s) may sound, for me they really were not after a while. When I have to eat or drink something every week it winds up tasting like medicine to me.

Since I have been asked for a smoothie recipe so many times in the past I will include what I used to use in mine (and I want to note that, for some reason unbeknownst to me, banana makes the smoothie far less effective. I don't know why though).

Quick(ish) Pineapple smoothie recipe:

Ingredients
- one whole (or half) pineapple)
- one yogurt (blueberry / vanilla work well)
- coconut water (or apple juice) – about 12oz (to taste)
- Optional: Blueberries or Strawberries
- Optional: approximately 4oz milk/cream/coffee-mate (coconut cream is pretty good in this too) -I put in cream or coffee-mate to help tackle the heartburn the citric acid in the pineapple gives me.

Instructions

Put contents into blender (with ice cubes if wanted) and blend for about a minute. Drink approximately 30 minutes prior to injecting (gradually finish as much as possible).

~~~~~~~~~~~~~~~

Now all of that said, I wanted to mention a few other medications. I did take a two-month "break" from Avonex back in 2000 to try out another medication called Rebif which is also a subcutaneous injection. The Rebif seems to work extremely well for many people but it didn't work well for me and after two months I went back to Avonex.

My Neurologist asked me if I had any interest in switching to a new oral medication called Gilenya but after reading about the side effects (i.e., reduced blood pressure, making the user more prone to infection, etc.) I decided to stay with

Avonex. As with the other meds, I know of many patients who have truly benefited from Gilenya but I was too scared to try it. At this time, there was another medication being studied called BG12 (from Biogen, the same company that makes Avonex) that sounded very promising. This is another pill and, while it would be a brand new medication for MS patients, it has been around for years in the UK (and has been used for years to treat psoriasis).

There are other oral medications in the works, but BG12 (AKA Tecfidera) is the one I'm most interested in. I know there is another one with a similar projected release date but, when I read that it had a 10% likelihood to cause hair loss, I decided against it (one side effect from the Avonex that I forgot to mention is how thin my hair has become. I believe that at least some of the hair thinning is from the Avonex. I don't know for sure, but I hope and pray to someday get my "normal" hair back even though I realize it may be too late for that to happen).

I should also mention that most of the medications I have just written about are for people with relapsing remitting Multiple Sclerosis. I don't know what is available for other forms of the disease (Benign, Primary Progressive, Secondary-Progressive, Malignant and/or Chronic Progressive

(NMSS. 2013)) but I hope and pray medications are in the works for MS patients in these categories as well. I believe things like liberation therapy for people who have Chronic Cerebrospinal Venous Insufficiency (CCSVI) and/or stem cell treatment may be helpful for more progressive forms of the condition. Please consult with your medical provider if you wish to learn more about this.

One thing that I take is not considered to be "real medicine" in many parts of this country. It is called Low Dose Naltrexone (also known as LDN). It really boggles my mind that it hasn't been approved as something that can be prescribed by doctors here - my hospital does not recognize it, unfortunately. There are some States where you can get a script written for it and there are Neurologists who you can get in touch with (online or by phone) to get the prescription. I have been on it since October of 2010 and it has helped me tremendously. It also appears to have a cumulative affect, meaning that over time it has made me feel better and better (and that different types of improvements keep happening to this day). I have had so many pain problems that at one point I had a running script of Oxycodone with Acetaminophen (sorry for not giving the drug name away. I don't want to be sued). I believe the pain became far worse when I developed Fibromyalgia, which I had diagnosed by a rheumatologist in 2010. Since I have been taking LDN I haven't had to take a single narcotic pain medication (thank goodness). I have found that, if the pain ever gets really bad, a Tramadol (2) seems to work for me (even though I wake up feeling like I've been hit by a truck the next day - so overwhelmingly tired. I can't tell if the main culprit for that is the pain or the meds or a combination of everything).

I am going to tell you my perception of what LDN is from what I've heard and what I've felt ever since I started taking it in October of 2010. Naltrexone is a substance that is (was?) used in the UK to help people end addictions to narcotics and alcohol. A low dose version of the drug has been affective for many people with a number of immunological disorders. The LDN turns down the brain's opioid receptors and, as a result, turns up endorphin production.

It is thought by many that LDN can help with cognitive function and fatigue. I haven't found the latter to be true (yet) but I agree that my cognitive functioning has improved. In addition, I haven't had to take any pain medications since I started using LDN. The pains are still with me, but they are nowhere near as bad as they were before taking the LDN. Bear in mind that I didn't start on LDN until after I was diagnosed with Fibromyalgia and after I spoke with my Neurologist to confirm it was safe to use while being on an MS Disease Modifying Drug (DMD). There have been other "perks" from the LDN that I don't want to get into here. Suffice it to say that the sexual "dysfunction" caused by anti-depressant drugs was a major problem for me until I had been on LDN for about six months; I go into more detail about this in the section "On a More Personal Note". There are videos in YouTube by people who have been, as they themselves have said, "saved" by LDN use.

LDN was recommended to my mother, who has Fibromyalgia, by another Fibro patient who takes it twice a day. Unfortunately, my mom tried it and she told me it didn't help her (again: different things work differently for different people). I found this to be understandable; my mother lives in constant pain and she prefers to go with what works best for her. I do not blame her for that at all. Being in that type of discomfort on an ongoing basis is not something she deserves and I think she has the right to go with whatever makes her most comfortable. As you continue living you will likely find yourself in the same "boat" as the rest of us. You will find things that work for you that don't for others and vise versa. We are our own best doctors at times, in my opinion.

Update (Friday, August 9, 2013): I am now in my fourth week of being un-medicated and waiting for this medication (Tecfidera/BG12) to arrive. The delay is because of my insurance company refusing to cover the medication.

Update 2 (Tuesday, November 25, 2013): The current list of Disease Modifying Drugs that are currently FDA approved and are available for people with relapsing remitting (and secondary progressive with continual relapses) forms of MS in the United States are as follows:

Aubagio (teriflunomide)
Avonex (interferon beta-1a)
Betaseron (interferon beta-1b)
Copaxone (glatiramer acetate)
Extavia (interferon beta-1b)
Gilenya (fingolimod)
Novantrone (mitoxantrone)

Rebif (interferon beta-1a)
Tecfidera (dimethyl fumarate)
Tysabri (natalizumab)
(NMSS 2013)

NOTE: The above medication list can be viewed on the National Multiple Sclerosis Society's web page at:

http://tinyurl.com/kughzno

Update 3 (Monday, November 25, 2013): I have been on Tecfidera for a little over three months now and I LOVE it. What I love about Tecfidera most is that it is a pill (not an injection) and the side effects are tolerable for me so I have my weekends back. I also love the way it is helping me feel better (i.e., the "muddle headed" feeling I used to have all the time is gone, I can feel my hands again, my headaches don't last as long, etc.). I will definitely write about this in much more detail in my next book. I just felt the need to mention it because I don't want to leave anybody "hanging" about how I have been doing on this new medicine.

On a More Personal Note

In this next section, I am going to go over a few topics that some may feel wade into "uncomfortable territory". There is some adult material following so if you are prone to taking offense, now is your chance to stop reading and move on to another section. I promise you, if "taboo" topic(s) bother you then something here will probably offend you (if not for what it says then for the fact that I had the audacity to bring it up). I will not get graphic, but I am going to go over a few issues that people sometimes have strong reactions to. Once again; if you are offended and/or bothered by discussions about sex, religion and/or politics now is your chance to pass on reading this section. If you continue to read this part of the book despite my warning please know that my intention is not to make people angry (and bear in mind that you have been warned).

The first thing I want to cover is sex. Since I was put on Anti-depressants during the first few years after I was diagnosed with MS, my sex drive was completely wiped out. I blame an SSRI Antidepressant Drug for that (as well as blaming one of the SSRIs for making me very jumpy, anxious and easy to startle. I have never gotten over that). I will refrain from naming the medication, but the bottle of pills for it listed "sexual side effects" as a commonly reported side effect. The antidepressant I was prescribed made me feel like a zombie. It completely dried me up and made me not care about anything or anyone, including myself. I was only on this medication for about a year, and it took almost 15 years for me to start getting any libido back. Of course, having had (very close to emergency) surgery to remove Fibroids did not help my libido much either.

In addition to the problem I was having from being on an anti-depressant, I am sure that having at least one UTI a month contributed to the lack of sexual desire. At the same time, however, I think the medication was much more influential. As for the "replenishment" of my libido I THINK it returned (at least in part) due to me using Low Dose Naltrexone (LDN).

I am very fortunate to have a husband who was completely patient and tolerant of my (just about) completely dead sex drive for so long. I know it did not make him happy (it certainly did not help me. I wanted to want sex but I had no interest in it at all). Thankfully my husband never forced me to do anything I did not want to do. He respects (and respected) me far too much to do that.

There are things that I can truly enjoy and appreciate now that I never enjoyed (because they caused me physical discomfort). One example of this is oral sex; even before the MS "reared its ugly head" this was something I never got any pleasure from.

I remember years ago, before I lived in Massachusetts (the first time I attempted to be a college student), when I had a boyfriend tell me there must have been something "biologically" wrong with me after I told him I was not interested in it. I remember being a bit taken aback and a little offended by this but now it appears he may have actually been right (even though to this day I think it was extremely rude of him to put me down for not liking something that he wanted to do to me). The ex-boyfriend I complain about in other sections was not the best boyfriend I have ever had, but he was much better than the "man" I was involved with in school who said this to me.

Once again, I think the LDN is what helped out with this as well as with giving me my libido back. I am nowhere near as active as I was before the MS manifested itself, but it is nice to at least be able to get some enjoyment out of sex and not to have to "fake it". Many people may read this and wonder why I am so convinced that the LDN is the reason for getting at least a part of my sex drive back. My reason for believing this is partly a process of elimination. I really have tried many, many different things that I had hoped would help (exercise, lotions, toys, books, films, etc.) and absolutely nothing else helped at all. I gave up hope after a while to be honest. The other reason I think it is the LDN is because I had read that LDN can lead to an increase in the production of endorphins.

When I first started looking into whether or not LDN might help me or not, I was sent a video made by someone who has MS and which can be viewed on YouTube at: http://tinyurl.com/k4hl7pm While looking at this video (and the two that follow it) I also discovered that LDN was thought to be helpful for people who had MS and/or Fibromyalgia (and other autoimmune conditions, including but not limited to Crohn's, Shingles, etc.). Like everything else, however, LDN works really well for some people and does absolutely nothing for others. My mother tried it out and it did nothing except make her uncomfortable.

I started the LDN very gradually. I use(d) distilled water to dissolve the pills in. When I started the treatment in October of 2010, I started with one Milliliter (Ml) per night. I read that it was ideal to do in the evening so I set a daily calendar event to remind me to take it every night at ten in the evening. I also had heard that the taste was awful (and it was/is - incredibly bitter) so I got some "fruit20" to mix with it for the first night. I did not care for the mix at all (and I avoid sugar substitutes as much as I can – fake sugar makes my head hurt very badly) so I kept experimenting until I found what worked best for me. I use a plastic dropper and I just take the LDN with the distilled water in a "straight shot" from the dropper. I then immediately drink a little bit of coffee (I find that kills the taste for me). I gradually worked my way up to and stopped at three ml per evening.

As far as the benefits of using LDN are concerned, I found them to be quite gradual and cumulative (as in the affects were and continue to be more diverse and better with time). It has been about three years since I first went on LDN and I have not felt the need to take an oxycodone since I started (a good thing, since the LDN might render a medication like that to be ineffective).

I wanted to very briefly go into the subject of spirituality and how I have used it to help me cope with getting this diagnosis, along with helping me with life in general. I am not going to try to preach or to convert anyone; I respect other peoples' opinions and beliefs as long as they respect mine. I am not a believer of any organized religion. I do not believe any of us has any way of knowing what is going to happen to us when we die, but I also believe there has to be some higher being or purpose somewhere. I do not appreciate it when someone preaches to me in the hopes of converting me and I have no intention of doing that to you.

I did go to Catholic school when I was a child (after my parents split up). I am a very rebellious person and, since my mother's side of the family is Jewish, my maternal grandmother once told me I was Jewish whether I "liked it or not." Not a very good thing to say to someone like me. I think I became Catholic just to spite what she said (and the notion that I was something that I did not believe in really bothered me. At the time I thought the word

It's Not as Bad as it Sounds

"Jewish" meant religious beliefs and didn't think of it as a culture). I wish this had not happened, looking back. Then again, while I wouldn't go back into my childhood for all the money in the world, I have to admit that the Catholic schools I attended were much more challenging (intellectually) to me than the public school I attended for my Senior year of high school. I am not saying that the teachers were better but I am sure all of the money they (the private school) got from the students and their families (with things like private tuition, mandatory "cookie sales" that all the students did twice a year, etc.) helped the Parochial school outshine the underfunded pubic school I graduated from. I do not think that is fair at all. I do not believe you should come from money to get a decent education, but I digress.

For years during and after I went to my first college in upstate New York, I honestly did not know what to say I was or what I truly believed in from a religious and/or spiritual perspective. For a long time, I told people I was Agnostic and that I did not believe in organized religion. I had and still have a problem with anything that teaches that people who don't follow it are "hell-bound". I had one teacher (a nun in my Parochial high school) who got very tired of me and asked me to stay out of her class. She felt my constant questions such as "why does the bible teach us that our pets will not go to

Heaven?" were a disruption to her students. She and I had an argument in the hallway one day and, when she saw she did not intimidate me, she got flustered and asked me to stay out of her class in exchange for giving me a B grade. I was more than happy to oblige.

Years after all of this and after finding out I had MS, I had a work colleague recommend a book to me (Thich Nhat Hạnh's Peace is Every Step: The Path of Mindfulness in Everyday Life). His reason for telling me about the book was not to "convert" me into any particular religion. He was telling me about how he used what he learned from this book to avoid having the anxiety attacks he was prone to. I got the book and it really changed my life. I had always been interested in learning about Buddhism and this book (and author, who I have read more by since), taught me a lot. Bear in mind that I had looked into other things that sparked my interest. One thing I had developed an interest in was Paganism and Wicca. I tried reading a few books on this but I did not find anything that really moved me.

I wound up developing my own spiritual code, so to speak. I still have my own way of doing things (I guess I could be considered a "solitary practitioner") and I see no reason to change. I am definitely not an Atheist. I believe there is something out there and I consider it to be a higher power. Other than that, I do not think it is within my capability to know what is "beyond" us in this life.

I bring up my spiritual beliefs and Thich Nhat Hanh because another thing I have found to be very helpful aside from eating well and exercising is meditation. When I first started getting into meditation, I had no idea what I was doing. I also had no idea this was something I could incorporate into my own daily practice(s). Many of the books I read about this in the past left me thinking it was much more structured than I believe it needed to be. This is something that I have chosen to do in a way that works for me. I realize that this is not something everyone will feel comfortable doing and, at the same time, may not hold the same benefits for people as it does for me. As I have stated over and over again throughout this writing, I am just mentioning what I like in the event that someone might try it and find it works for them as well.

The last item I am going to (VERY briefly) go over is politics. Do not worry – I won't stay on this subject for too long. I am not going to try to sway anyone's' viewpoints here either. I know what a "hot spot" this topic is and I am also not going to tell you my political beliefs or who I voted for. I guess all I want to say here is that, when and if you get involved in doing anything political, you need to develop a very thick skin since this is a topic that makes people angrier than I ever could have imagined in the past.

In the same way that reading some things online may really scare someone about a health condition, reading peoples' political views online can be nerve wracking (and/or anger inducing). I made the mistake of looking up something a politician said today. I didn't agree with what he had to say, and then I made the mistake of reading the message board underneath his statements. I really regret doing this; I got so upset and so angry that I gave myself a horrible headache. It is definitely possible to accidentally make yourself feel worse if you let yourself get too upset/angry/stressed out over something you read. Additionally, if you leave angry responses to things that bother you be prepared to get worse in return. Some people love getting others all worked up – they thrive on it. It is not worth risking your health over.

Now I am going to move on to some more sections for the book. I know I only "delved" into this particular topic. If you want to read more about this, please let me know via email (ydcbook@gmail.com). I plan to write another book (or two) based at least partially on feedback I get from this one. I am eager to see what types of

It's Not as Bad as it Sounds

things we have in common because, as I discovered with Stan's MS Angels (www.stansangels.com) and other online support groups, a lot of us have very similar back stories.

How Did This Start And Where Did Things Go?

(i.e., before the diagnosis;

day-to-day symptoms)

As I begin this section, I am once again thinking of the questions I had when I first learned I had MS. Please be aware that you will probably see quite a few similarities between this section and the section called My Exacerbations & Experiences (these chapters were written about two years apart from each other and I apologize if this causes any confusion).

It's Not as Bad as it Sounds

When I went to see the Rheumatologist who diagnosed me with Fibro I went to him for confirmation as I already suspected I had it. I was, therefore, completely prepared for the diagnosis. Finding out I had MS, on the other hand, was earth shattering. I had not done any significant research into the condition and I did not know enough about it. Finding out I had it terrified me because I thought of worst-case scenarios I had read and/or heard about/saw.

A major unknown for me was what to expect in the future (both near and distant). Unfortunately, MS makes expecting just about anything difficult. One of the problems I have always had with it was and continues to be not knowing what to expect from one day or one moment to the next.

I am going to start with what happened to bring me to the Hospital to get my unofficial diagnosis - the one I received the year prior to the "official DX" (i.e., the one I chose to ignore since things were left "up in the air" and since the doctors could not tell me precisely what was wrong with me). I had some health issues leading up to the diagnosis that were fairly strong indicators that there was a bigger health problem than I was aware of at that time. I was in my mid-twenties and still felt like a "young adult." One problem that first presented itself and gradually got worse was getting diagnosed with urinary tract infections (UTIs). I remember thinking I was being punished by some "higher power" for having sex without being married; it reached a point where I was getting at least one UTI every month and the UTIs just kept getting more and more painful.

One side note with regards to the UTIs (this is something that I debated putting into the section about people who (should) have their feet in their mouths): my ex-boyfriend took me to a hospital in an area near his home and the doctor who saw me was horrible with people, or at least he was with me. He actually asked me "how I wiped" when I "pee-peed" (and/or "pooed"). These were his words, not mine. He also showed me a photo of a man and asked if I found him attractive. I was a bit offended and a little shaken by this. My boyfriend was right there with me, I was in a world of pain due to a UTI and this man was trying to get me to say I was attracted to someone he had a picture of. I finally gave a very non-committal "yeah he's ok I guess." The Doctor then all too happily informed me that the man in the picture had Aids. He then suggested that, whenever I had intercourse, I should use at least two condoms.

This same unpleasant-to-deal with Doctor then catheterized me to see if he could determine what was happening. I don't know if all of the readers of this know what being catheterized involves, but if you are aware I think you will agree with me that this Doctor was probably as rude as he was because he knew I was going to be completely vulnerable when he catheterized me. For anyone who does not know what it is - it involves placing a tube into a body cavity to allow for passage of fluid (The American Heritage® Dictionary. 2003).

That was an incredibly inappropriate and bad way to deal with a patient as well as very poorly timed. The Doctor was unable to do anything except give me antibiotics and I was very happy to leave his hospital after that. Unfortunately, the UTIs just kept happening over and over again. It seemed that the only way to avoid getting an infection was to avoid intercourse altogether. If I had known then that I had MS I would have known why I was getting so many UTIs. I now have a Urologist and have thankfully learned ways to avoid getting UTIs (most of the time).

A short time after this happened I started having trouble breathing (I would wheeze whenever I inhaled). I had a Saturday night to Sunday morning visit with my ex-boyfriend. The breathing problems happened while I was at his home so I stayed at his place for an extra night. On Monday, he took me to a train station so I could go back into the city I live in to go to a good hospital. I told him I never wanted to go to the one where I had the awful UTI experience again. I went to a well-known Hospital's emergency room and was given (temporarily) an oxygen inhaler. After being seen I was told I had bronchitis and that, if I did not quit smoking cigarettes, it would become chronic. I was given an asthma inhaler and told I should quit smoking. I go into more detail on other medical issues I had in the section My Multiple Sclerosis (and Fibromyalgia) "Journey".

Since I have covered the odd medical issues I had leading up to my diagnosis, I now want to go over some of the day-to-day symptoms and side effects that I experience. I need you to keep something in mind though; MS is different for everyone. I do not think I can stress that enough. I once heard MS compared to snowflakes because each case varies so much. Much like the medical condition itself, different medications affect different patients in different ways.

I currently use Avonex (one of the "CRAB" (Copaxone, Rebif, Avonex, and Betaseron) drugs. I know many people who tried to use these medications and who had such strong reactions to them that they had to stop. I also know of others who refused to medicate until something came out in pill form. I cannot fault anyone for being unwilling and/or unable to give themselves injections/shots. I was astounded (as was my mother) that I was able to perform injections on myself at all. I believe the reason I could was because my fear of what the MS could do to me was much worse than my fear of needles. That fear drove me to force myself to self-inject and to pretend and/or convince myself it did not bother me.

Once again, I want to make it clear that my MS may not be anything like yours (if you have it) or anyone you know who has it if you do not. I do not want you to be alarmed if you are going through anything you do not see discussed in this chapter and/or book. Just know this – you are not alone. In addition, please know that some of my day-to-day problems are from the Fibromyalgia (and sometimes I don't know whether the MS or the Fibro is the main cause of the problem).

One of my worst MS (and/or Fibro) symptoms is fatigue. I am listing that one first because I never feel awake/energetic. I am thankful that I never (or almost never) have bouts of insomnia but it would be lovely to feel alert for a change. Before I was diagnosed ("officially") I remember getting very tired and going to bed at eight o'clock one night. I slept until five the following afternoon, and the only reason I woke up was because my phone was ringing. Twenty-one hours of sleep may sound good to some who read this but it was not good at all. I find I feel worse if I oversleep than I do if I do not sleep enough and this was no exception – I felt like I had lost a boxing match or something.

Another issue I have is with my short-term memory (and long-term in some cases. I don't remember a thing about my sophomore year of high school – it is a literal black hole in my memory). My memory problems started happening while I was still in my twenties so I am unconvinced that the memory gaps are all "age-related". I know of many other MS Patients who have the same problem. Fibromyalgia can cause cognitive troubles too (known as "Fibro

Fog"). I wouldn't be surprised if the combination of MS and Fibro make the cognitive troubles worse and the same is true about the fatigue.

Now I want to go over pain problems. Pain is a daily reality. Some of the pain is from the MS. I used to get migraines constantly when I was in high school. I get "regular" headaches almost every day now. These headaches are probably a result of both the MS and the Fibro. Some of the pains and/or tenderness are from the Fibro. Another part of the pain and/or discomfort is a left over residual symptom from one of the worst MS attacks I ever had (when my left arm went numb and I couldn't use it (I'm left handed) for about a month). After I was treated for this attack, I got use of my arm back but both my left and right hands now have a level of numbness, tingling and/or pain to them that I have had to learn to live with. I'm not happy about it but it is life. My mantra is (still) that, as long as I can walk unassisted, I am happy.

I try to stay positive as much as I possibly can because when I am feeling unwell and/or downhearted my outlook tends to go downhill. My general experience has been that being negative gets me nowhere. It actually leads me into depression, which just makes my fatigue more pronounced. This is a vicious cycle because, if I don't go to sleep when I should and I allow myself to get too fatigued, my outlook goes downhill and I start to feel a lot worse.

After the attack was "cleared up" (not with Steroids as I have a bad reaction to them, but by infusions of Immunoglobulin) a new pain problem started to develop. I started having horrible spasms in my back. Initially this did not happen very often, thankfully. I am glad it did not because it scared both my husband and me. The spasm attack lasted for hours and I was in so much pain I could not do anything except roll around on a hardwood floor in the hopes of getting the pain to stop.

It's Not as Bad as it Sounds

I called my Neurologist's office the following day. Since she is part of an MS clinic, I was able to get helped pretty quickly. I was told that the pains I was experiencing were "spasticity" pains and I was given a prescription for a mild muscle relaxant. I was very nervous about taking the muscle relaxant but I was assured that the dose was extremely low. I gave in and decided to give the medication a try. I still take it now (in the evening) in the hopes of making the spasms occur less frequently.

Other day-to-day issues I deal with run the gamut. I have a tremor (that I was born with, according to my mother). If I get a little nervous my "mild" tremor turns into a very pronounced shake, leading others around me to think I'm nervous, scared or "over excited" about things. It is incredibly frustrating. I am glad high school is long past. I remember a teacher giving me a "D" grade for a speech because, as she said herself when I questioned the bad grade, my "knees were shaking". Not a really good reason to give a student a D, in my opinion. It is also a bit embarrassing to have my shake pointed out to me (as if it was something I was not aware of). Guess this is just another case of people not thinking before they speak. Having my tremor pointed out to me just makes me feel a little more insecure over the fact that my shake is being watched (which can make the shake more pronounced – another vicious cycle).

I believe I also have "drop foot" (or "foot drop") because of the odd way my shoes wear away (and constant comments about how I "walk funny" and/or drag my feet). I do not think it is that bad yet but, if it ever does become unmanageable, I know there are ways to treat it. I believe that some of the ways to treat drop foot are non-medicinal. Since I currently take so many pills I would prefer a non-medicalized approach to whatever I can take. I have a month long pill planner that I have split into two sections: night pills and morning pills. I hate it but it is the only way I can be certain that I don't forget to take anything I need. I also have a card that I carry in my purse listing all of the medications I am currently on. I did this because I know whenever I have a doctor appointment I will be asked what I take. Not being able to write without it hurting inspired me to make a pill card. I have some trouble with walking up and down stairs due to pain in my knees too. This pain could be from the Fibro, the MS or just from overuse.

Once again, I often have a hard time figuring out which condition (or syndrome) is the "culprit" for what I am feeling. Although, if and when the pain is a Fibro pain, whatever area hurts feels worse when touched directly. I do not think MS pains work the same way since I believe the pains are (misdirected?) signals coming from the brain The Fibromyalgia "trigger points" and areas around them, however, are extremely sensitive to touch, particularly during spasms.

I am also very dry-mouthed on an almost constant basis. There are a number of symptoms that result from the medications an MS and/or Fibro patients might take. Symptoms including, but not limited to dehydration, fatigue, depression and cognitive difficulties can arise from both prescription and over the counter medications along with the way they interact with each other.

One other item I wanted to bring up here involves looking for a job for anyone who has MS (or Fibro, or a host of other disabilities/syndromes/etc.) and the issue I am focusing on is whether or not it is a good idea to disclose about your illness. I no longer do this when I am being interviewed because I do not want to scare away a potential employer. I had a position at a University that may not have been as horrible as it was if I had been able to tell my boss I had MS. Unfortunately, I had been laid off from another job because of the MS so I did not think it would be a wise thing to mention and I was right in many but (possibly) not all cases.

It's Not as Bad as it Sounds

It infuriates me that we have to keep our health conditions a secret in order to avoid missing out on employment opportunities as if we are to blame for our illnesses. The idea that a company will not hire someone if they find out he or she has a disability certainly seems like discrimination to me. I have decided at this point in my life that, if someone will not agree to let me work for or with them because I have MS, they are not worthy of my time and/or consideration and I want nothing to do with them.

I am convinced that I am missing out on "opportunities" because of this but I am appalled that we have to lie about something we have no control over just to get work. For those of us with "invisible disabilities", the need for special accommodations can lead to not being able to find and/or retain employment. For many of us, our day-to-day symptoms are visible to others. This can make finding employment (and remaining employed) almost impossible.

The Things I'm Grateful For

Now I want to take some time to discuss some of the "perks" that I have discovered since being diagnosed (first with Multiple Sclerosis and then with Fibromyalgia). I know that may be a somewhat irritating sentence to read, but good things have come out of this and I would be remiss if I didn't mention any of them.

I want to start by writing about an online support group for people who have MS that I have found to be incredibly helpful. It is called "Stan's Angels".

The URL for the group is http://www.stansangels.com/. The person who started it is Stan Swartz and I was fortunate enough to join when he had just put the support group together so he and I have become very good friends. If I had not discovered his web page, I honestly do not think I would have come out of the diagnosis with the healthy attitude and/or outlook I have now. I also do not think I would have ever thought to write this book without his support page.

Stan started the group when he was working with Dr. Timothy Vollmer. Dr. Vollmer is a friend of Stan's and was formerly the head of Neurology at

It's Not as Bad as it Sounds

Barrow Neurological Institute. He has since been promoted to another position.

I have made some very strong friendships on Stan's page. I have also received wonderful and helpful advice and, best of all, it is a great place to go and vent to others who I know understand where I am coming from. One of the not-so-great things about MS and Fibro (among other physical problems) is that, by being "invisible disabilities", these conditions lead to a lot of trouble with making the rest of the world believe that we have (serious) problems and that those problems are not within our control.

Yvonne Decelis

I am constantly reading about people who have
friends, family members, partners, etc. who do not
see that they are sick and therefore don't
understand why they can't do things a "normal
person" could do. They cannot see that something is
wrong with us and therefore assume that we are
fine (and that we are being unreasonable, uncaring
or lazy, etc.) I have written a "side note" to all
friends, family members and loved ones of people
who have these "invisible" illnesses at the end of
the section My MS (and Fibro) "Journey" if you ever
need to show it to someone.

This leads to a lot of problems for us and it was
really wonderful to find a web page where I knew

people would understand exactly what I was talking about. At the same time, this is a support group that I didn't find to be overwhelmingly negative and/or depressing. One thing you will hear a lot if you have a disability is that stress (and/or negativity) should be avoided at all costs. We know how impossible that advice is to follow and it would certainly help us out a lot if we didn't have to constantly defend ourselves to the rest of the world. We are not lazy, stupid, uncaring (or any of the other incredibly hurtful things people call us) and we should not have to prove ourselves to anyone.

We (the Angels) watch out for each other and support each other as much as we possibly can. I have seen Angels turn to each other for advice on a wide spectrum of things. One thing that comes up often is that we give each other online support when someone is having an attack, when someone is in a situation where they aren't being treated fairly, or giving each other advice on things like how to collect disability. In addition, even though this is an online support group some of the Angels have met up with each other in real life (and a few actually got married).

Another item I want to bring up is collecting Disability benefits (SSDI) from Social Security. Applying for and getting Disability is not an easy task at all. Saying it is very time-consuming is an understatement. If you try to apply for disability directly through your Social Security office, do not be shocked if and when you get rejected. I believe almost everyone is rejected initially which I suppose is understandable considering our government probably does not want (nor can they afford) to give money to everyone and anyone who comes looking for it.

My advice is that you should not try to do this alone. Also, do not try to act and/or look healthier than you are. A lot of us make that mistake; I certainly did and it worked against me. It took me almost three years to get approved for SSDI and, had I not tried so hard to make myself seem completely normal, I probably would have gotten it a lot sooner. In addition, I used a Disability Law Group after getting three rejections. I should have gone to the Disability Law Group after the first rejection but was not aware of this at the time.

The upside of working with the law group was that they eventually won the case for me and only charged twenty-five percent of the back pay (i.e., the amount of money collected from SSDI during the time from when one first applies to when they are accepted) I received from SS. The downside was that it took an extremely long time to get approved and that I really could have used that extra twenty-five percent. If you don't win, they don't charge anything.

Since I did this I have learned that, depending on income eligibility and local rules and regulations, going through my local Federal Congress people would have probably been faster and would have saved me the money that I wound up paying the law group who won my disability case. It also would have probably helped me avoid the inexplicable delay in getting my back pay (the law group was not able to help me with this so I ended up having an elected official help me get the back pay).

Collecting Disability allowed me to quit two part time jobs I was unhappy doing and also gave me the ability to go back to school full time. I often hear people telling me that getting laid off was "the best thing that ever happened" to them. (NOT something you want and/or need to hear immediately after getting laid off and/or let go).

It took a long time (from 2006 to almost 2012) but I am finally able to say it to myself and/or others. I honestly don't think I would have been able to get my Bachelors' degree (as well as get two certifications, make the Dean's list and then go on to Graduate school) if it hadn't been for me losing my full time job and eventually getting SSDI.

It's Not as Bad as it Sounds

Do I plan to stay on Disability forever? I am hoping the answer to that will be "no" but it is impossible to know what is going to happen with a disease like Multiple Sclerosis. I am not a fan of Fibromyalgia (which causes me pain, "Fibro fog", and fatigue) but I don't believe it is anywhere near as degenerative a condition as MS can be. I could be wrong about that however; remember – I am a patient not a medical professional.

The next item I want to discuss is exercise and "healthful" living. It took me a very long time to get over finding out I had MS and the first few years after the diagnosis did not go very well for me.

During this time, I got out of one relationship and into another and I also had bad luck with the first medication I was given. In 1999, however, Montel Williams was diagnosed and he donated money to a hospital I now use (Brigham and Women's' - http://brighamandwomens.org/) so that they could open up their own MS clinic.

I did quite a bit of research on what was going on with Montel and discovered that he used exercise to help promote his well-being. I was already exercising and trying to be healthy but, until finding out about how well it worked for him, I had no idea what a huge difference exercise could make for me. I quit smoking (not easy at all), quit drinking diet soda (even harder than quitting smoking, much to my surprise), and started eating less junk food and more vegetables and fruits (also not easy and very expensive). As for the exercise; it was not easy to get into in the beginning. I hated it for about a year, to be perfectly honest.

I am very fortunate that athleticism runs in my family. Even though I was never athletic as a child, I became quite athletic as a result of my workout routine. I am still as active as I can be. I also am in a study being conducted at Tufts Medical School on the effects of Tai Chi on people who have Fibromyalgia. This is a six-month study and I am currently halfway through it. I can honestly say that Tai Chi has helped me out quite a bit (as has my instructor, Ramel Rones).

I would like to include some information about Ramel's training here since he has videos and books you can buy at Amazon. He also has a class you can take online at Udemy (https://www.udemy.com/). If you go to Ramel's home page the best discount you can get for his class is available there: www.ramelrones.com. I took and recommend his Sunset Tai Chi training. You do not have to be an athlete to do this – it is intended for beginners so please do not be afraid to give it a try if you are curious about it.

It's Not as Bad as it Sounds

Another item I am very happy about is having the opportunity to be a "Commonwealth Diversity Fellowship" participant. This was a program launched by the college I attended in 2010. I was in the "first batch" of participants for the program. This involved doing a Fellowship for a State agency.

I wound up getting my Fellowship in the Department of Veteran Services (DVS). This confused me a little bit initially because I was a Gerontology (i.e., the study of aging) major which led me to think I would be put in the office for Elder Affairs. I was initially very confused and worried about this placement decision but it did not take long before I recognized the value of it.

Since the semester I was assigned to this Fellowship I have stayed on. Not only did I figure out why I was put into this department, I found that I had very strong feelings about the type of work I was being asked to do (involving helping Veterans find employment and/or volunteer opportunities) and that I had quite a bit of empathy for the Veterans that work(ed) with this office.

In addition to learning a lot about Veterans, I learned much about Post Traumatic Stress as well as about conflicts in other countries (and the people who have gone overseas to fight for our safety). The woman I report to in the Department of Veteran Services (DVS) pointed out that she does not like the "D" in the acronym PTSD. Her reasoning for this is that if it is considered a "disorder" it can be too easily dismissed (by doctors, counselors, etc.) but if it is looked on as an "Injury" then professionals will be more likely to treat the Veterans who have it instead of just dismissing them as having "mental problems". Based on things I have seen, such as the documentary "Wartorn: 1861-2010" a very hard (for me) to watch but extremely moving documentary, I agree with her.

There is a group who report to this office called the SAVE team. To quote the DVS web page, the Statewide Advocacy for Veterans' Empowerment (SAVE) has the following mission: "'You Give Us the Call...We'll Give You the Answer.'

The fundamental principle of the SAVE program is to advocate for veterans who are not able to obtain the benefits they have earned due to institutional or personal barriers. The program's primary mission is prevention of suicide and mental health distress through the identification of issues facing veterans when they return from service and proactively providing them with access to benefits and services that may address these issues and

result in positive transitions back to civilian life."
(DVS 2008)

I was privileged enough to watch a training by one
of the SAVE Team Veterans called
"BATTLEMIND". If you want to learn more please
check out the webinar version of Battlemind (you
will need Quick time on whatever browser you wish
to view/listen to this on): http://tinyurl.com/kpfbsc5

One other interesting thing that has come out of
this was discovering a common bond with many of
the Veterans that I have come across while working
with this office. I have had a few Veterans ask me if
I would consider giving talks on getting through

dealing with people not understanding why those with invisible pain act the way they do. I was very moved and honored by this request (and it is an avenue I would love to explore, health problems notwithstanding.)

Odds and Ends

Conclusion

Now that you have read this book, I truly hope you are able to come away from it having learned something to help you and/or people you know. I am using this last section for a few miscellaneous "odds and ends" and to leave you with some contact information.

One other item I wanted to go over was the idea of using Cannabis as medication. I know (from experience) that using Cannabis helps with appetite and with depression but I feel it also can help make certain types of pain, such as the "MS hug" tolerable. Is it something I think should be legal? Absolutely! I do not understand why it still is not, to be honest. I suppose I should say I suspect one of the primary reasons it still is not legal is greed. I am also of the opinion that "alternative therapies" (including, but not limited to Homeopathic and/or Holistic Medicine, Reflexology, Reiki, Acupuncture, etc.) can be very helpful to many people. I am not convinced that the "Medical System" is the only hope we have to have good health and/or a good quality of life.

It's Not as Bad as it Sounds

I am now going to include my latest "soap-box" rant about why I think Cannabis is not legal in the United States. I wrote this years ago for a Legalization web page: the (main) reasons pot is not legal is because of William Randolph Hearst (the "paper baron" who, back in the early 20th century, owned a communication empire - newspapers, land that was timber property. He had stock in every facet of the production of his newspapers and didn't want to compete with anything else. The fact that he was mega-wealthy did not hurt because as we know, the "all mighty dollar" means so much in this country) and because of racism against Blacks and Hispanics. So for those of you who put us down and accuse us of being bad examples for our children: educate yourselves before you start throwing stones. You've allowed yourself to be manipulated by a broken system and you don't know what you are talking about when you yell at us and call us druggies. It's just like calling marijuana a gateway drug. It isn't - if it was over 90% of the population would be checked into drug clinics. The war on drugs is a failure. A big, EXPENSIVE, corrupt failure!

OK – that is it for my Soap box. I now want to leave you with what I believe and hope could be some good contact information for you to have. I also want to leave you with the final thought that you are very likely to be capable of much more than you realize. Believe me, if I could get to where I am today, I think you have a very good shot at it too. I just wish I knew a long time ago what I know now. I never trusted my own abilities and I wound up paying for that. I think we all underestimate ourselves.

If you want to learn more, please feel free to contact me at YDCBook@yahoo.com. It may take me a while to get back to you but I will try my best. I thank you in advance for your understanding and patience! We (members of the disabled community) are all in this together. In my opinion, we can all really help each other out in more ways than many have ever dreamed possible.

Potentially Useful contact/information:

The National Multiple Sclerosis Society
http://www.nationalmssociety.org/index.aspx
National Offices:

New York
733 Third Ave.
3rd Floor
New York, NY 10017

Advocacy Office
1100 New York Ave.,N.W.
Suite 660
Washington, DC 20005

Denver
900 South Broadway
Suite 200
Denver, CO 80209

The Multiple Sclerosis Association of America
http://www.mymsaa.org/

National Headquarters
706 Haddonfield Road
Cherry Hill, NJ 08002
Toll-free: (800) 532-7667
Main Telephone: (856) 488-4500

**National Institute of Arthritis and
Musculoskeletal and Skin Diseases (NIAMS)**
http://www.niams.nih.gov/
Information Clearinghouse
National Institutes of Health
1 AMS Circle
Bethesda, MD 20892-3675
Phone: 301-495-4484
Toll Free: 877-22-NIAMS (877-226-4267)
TTY: 301-565-2966
Fax: 301-718-6366
Email: NIAMSinfo@mail.nih.gov
Website: http://www.niams.nih.gov

Stan's Angels
http://www.stansangels.com
Rocky Mountain MS Center
http://www.mscenter.org/
Rocky Mountain MS Center
8845 Wagner Street
Westminster, CO 80031

US House Of Representatives
(To find your local Representative online)
http://www.house.gov/representatives/find/

Homeopathic Medicine
http://www.webmd.com/balance/guide/homeopathy-topic-overview

A friend of mine who is a fellow Fibro patient recommended the following Homeopathic specialist. (I have not used this person's services but am leaving this contact information in as a courtesy):

www.rebeccaelmalehmd.com
Dr. Christine Hochhauser
(212) 253-2488

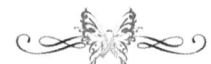

Index

Sources

"Catheter." *The American Heritage® Dictionary of the English Language, Fourth Edition.* 2003. Houghton Mifflin Company 26 Nov. 2013.

"Dosing That Fits Your Schedule." *Once-a-Week AVONEX.* Biogen, 2013. Web. 30 Nov. 2013.

"Fibromyalgia." *Questions and Answers About.* N.p., n.d. Web. 20 Nov. 2013.

"Google LDN ! Part One." *YouTube.* YouTube, 01 Jan. 2009. Web. 06 Dec. 2013.

Sources, continued

"LDN and Autoimmune Disease." *LDN and Autoimmune Disease.* N.p., n.d. Web. 20 Nov. 2013.

"Multiple Sclerosis." *Types of MS.* N.p., n.d. Web. 20 Nov. 2013.

"National Multiple Sclerosis Society." *About MS: National MS Society.* N.p., n.d. Web. 18 Nov. 2013.

"National Multiple Sclerosis Society." *Treatments: National MS Society.* N.p., n.d. Web. 24 Nov. 2013.

"Partners HealthCare®." *Physician Finder.* N.p., n.d. Web. 20 Nov. 2013.

It's Not as Bad as it Sounds

Sources, continued

"The Show Must Go On." *YouTube.* YouTube, 06 Dec. 2007. Web. 23 Nov. 2013.

"Statewide Advocacy for Veterans' Empowerment (SAVE)." *Statewide Advocacy for Veterans' Empowerment (SAVE).*

Commonwealth of Massachusetts, 7 Mar. 2008. Web. 27 Dec. 2013.

"Welcome to the Multiple Sclerosis Association of America." *MSAA: The Multiple Sclerosis Association Of America.* N.p., n.d. Web. 20 Nov. 2013

Wilbert, Caroline. "Fibromyalgia a 'Real Disease,' Study Shows." WebMD. WebMD, 2008. Web. 11 Nov. 2014.

www.ingramcontent.com/pod-product-compliance
Lightning Source LLC
Chambersburg PA
CBHW070636290526
45790CB00001B/108